100 FOODS

YOU DIDN'T KNOW YOU COULD EAT

Publications International, Ltd.

TABLE OF CONTENTS

FOODS YOU DIDN'T KNOW YOU COULD EAT

Many people with diabetes assume, especially when first diagnosed, that having the disease means cutting all the delicious, satisfying foods from their diet. Nothing could be further from the truth. There is no special "diabetic diet" anymore. While people with diabetes need to take special care in managing their blood sugar, they, their spouses or partners, and their families can all strive for a varied, heart-healthy diet that's full of tasty, colorful foods.

Foods that are most beneficial to people with diabetes are primarily minimally processed, or "whole foods," because they tend to be lower in calories and unhealthy fats. Additionally, these foods are superior because they contain higher amounts of naturally occurring nutrients. These can include fiber and other complex carbohydrates, protein, healthy fats, essential vitamins and minerals, and phytonutrients (plant nutrients). A growing body of research indicates these nutrients can aid in blood sugar control and help fight health problems associated with diabetes.

Many foods fit the bill, and *100 Foods You Didn't Know You Could Eat* is your guide to the top choices. Delicious foods that make the grade include dark chocolate, popcorn, oatmeal, peanut butter, raspberries, and shrimp. Read the food profiles to understand how each food can help people with diabetes. You'll also find tips on how to properly select, store, prepare, and serve each food to maintain the best quality, flavor, and health benefits. Several recipes are sprinkled throughout the book. Each recipe includes nutritional information and dietary exchanges.

WHAT ARE EXCHANGE LISTS?

To make it simple to add variety to meals, easy-to-use exchange lists are published. Exchange lists divide foods into categories, such as starches, fats, fruits, vegetables, meats, and so on, with predetermined portion sizes. All food exchanges within a category have roughly equivalent nutritional value and impact on blood sugar levels. For example, one starch exchange contains about 15 grams of carbohydrate, 3 grams of protein, and about 80 calories. If your meal plan calls for one starch exchange for breakfast, you can look at an exchange list to see that that's equivalent to a half cup of cereal, half of a frozen bagel, a half cup of cooked grits, or one slice of rye bread.

Exchange Group	Carbohydrate	Protein	Fat	Calories
1 Starch exchange	15g	3g	Trace	80
1 Fruit exchange	15g	None	None	60
1 Vegetable exchange	5g	2g	None	25
1 Milk exchange	12g	8g	1–8g	90–150
1 Meat exchange	None	7g	3–8g	35–100
1 Fat exchange	None	None	5g	45

ACORN SQUASH

This acorn-shaped variety of winter squash is full of flavor and nutrients. It's easy to find during fall and winter months and simple to prepare. It's most commonly baked, and its slightly sweet-tasting flesh is high in fiber.

BENEFITS:

Acorn squash is rich in vitamins A (beta-carotene) and C and the mineral potassium. Although acorn squash is a starchy vegetable, its high fiber content helps slow the rate that carbohydrates are digested and absorbed, making it a great choice for people with diabetes. Its high potassium level also makes it beneficial for controlling blood pressure.

HOW TO SELECT AND STORE:

You may find acorn squash year-round, but it's best from early fall to late winter. Look for acorn squash that is dark green with some golden coloring and free of spots, bruises, and mold. The hard skin serves as a barrier, allowing it to be stored a month or more in a dark, cool place.

NUTRIENTS PER SERVING:

Acorn squash, ½ cup cooked
Calories: 57
Protein: 1g
Total fat: 0g
Saturated fat: 0g
Cholesterol: 0mg
Carbohydrate: 15g
Dietary fiber: 4.5g
Sodium: 0mg
Potassium: 450mg
Calcium: 45mg
Iron: 9mg
Vitamin A: 439 IU
Vitamin C: 11mg
Folate: 19mcg

TIPS:

Acorn squash can be baked, steamed, sautéed, or simmered. One of the easiest cooking methods is to cut it in half, scoop out and discard the seeds, and bake it for about an hour. You can serve the baked squash in the skin and fill the center with whatever you like (try rice, barley, pine nuts, and garlic), or you can scoop out the baked flesh and enjoy it mashed or sprinkled with a small amount of Parmesan cheese or other seasonings. Acorn squash is also a tasty addition to savory soups.

GLAZED MAPLE ACORN SQUASH

1 large acorn or golden acorn squash

¼ cup water

2 tablespoons pure maple syrup

1 tablespoon margarine or butter, melted

¼ teaspoon ground cinnamon

NUTRIENTS PER SERVING:

Calories: 90
Protein: 1g
Total fat: 3g
Saturated fat: 0.5g
Cholesterol: 8mg
Carbohydrate: 18g
Dietary fiber: 2g
Sodium: 39mg
Dietary exchanges:
1 Starch, ½ Fat

1. Preheat oven to 375°F.

2. Cut stem and blossom ends from squash. Cut squash crosswise into 4 equal slices. Discard seeds and membrane. Place water in 13×9-inch baking dish. Arrange squash in dish; cover with foil. Bake 30 minutes or until tender.

3. Combine maple syrup, margarine, and cinnamon in small bowl; mix well. Uncover squash; pour off water. Brush squash with syrup mixture, letting excess pool in center of squash rings.

4. Bake 10 minutes or until syrup mixture is bubbly.

Makes 4 or 5 servings

ALMONDS

Although we call them nuts, almonds are actually the seeds of the fruit from an almond tree. We get a host of nutrients, most notably vitamin E, protein, and healthy, monounsaturated fat, when we munch on almond seeds.

BENEFITS:

Almonds pack a powerful nutrient punch in a small package. Their combination of protein, fiber, and healthy fats makes them a great food that provides lasting energy. They are an excellent source of vitamin E and magnesium and offer calcium and B vitamins, too. Almonds and other nuts are also known to help lower cholesterol levels. Because almonds are calorie-rich, portion control is important.

NUTRIENTS PER SERVING:

Almonds, 1 ounce dry roasted without salt
Calories: 169
Protein: 6g
Total fat: 15g
Saturated fat: 1g
Cholesterol: 0mg
Carbohydrate: 6g
Dietary fiber: 3g
Sodium: 0mg
Potassium: 200mg
Calcium: 76mg
Iron: 1mg
Folate: 15mcg
Vitamin E: 7mg
Magnesium: 80mg

HOW TO SELECT AND STORE:

Almonds are available packaged or in bulk, with or without shells. Always check the freshness date on packaged almonds. Packaged almonds are available in various forms—whole, blanched (to remove the skin), sliced, slivered, raw, dry or oil roasted, smoked, flavored, and salted or unsalted. Almonds in the shell can keep for a few months in a cool, dry location. Once you shell them or open a package of shelled nuts, they will need to be stored in the refrigerator or freezer.

TIPS:

Using almonds as a topping or in baking allows you to benefit from their nutrients without overdoing calories. As a snack, stick with a handful, or about 23 almonds (1 ounce). Dry roasted almonds are lower in calories than oil roasted. Enjoy unsalted almonds sprinkled on salads, soups, casseroles, vegetables, stir-fries, cereal, and more.

APPLES

With various colors and textures, chances are, you've tasted only a few of the thousands of apple varieties grown today. Apples are a great low-fat, fiber-packed food that can be enjoyed in many different ways.

BENEFITS:

Whether you snack on apple slices or add them to a salad, apples' versatility and nutrient content make them an excellent food to incorporate into your diet. They provide vitamin C, an antioxidant that may help prevent heart disease and some cancers. Their soluble fiber helps lower cholesterol and slows absorption of carbohydrates, which aids in evening out blood sugar levels.

HOW TO SELECT AND STORE:

A few varieties, such as Golden Delicious, Jonathan, and Winesap, are all-purpose apples. But in general, choose apples for their intended purposes. For baking, try Empire, Rome Beauty, Cortland, or Northern Spy. They deliver flavor and keep their shape when cooked. For eating raw, you can't beat Gala, Fuji, Braeburn, or Honeycrisp. Apples prefer humid air, so your refrigerator's crisper drawer is the best place for storage. Some varieties will keep for several months, but most get mealy within a month or two.

NUTRIENTS PER SERVING:

Apple, 1 medium
Calories: 95
Protein: <1g
Total fat: 0g
Saturated fat: 0g
Cholesterol: 0g
Carbohydrate: 25g
Dietary fiber: 4g
Sodium: 0mg
Potassium: 195mg
Calcium: 11mg
Vitamin A: 98 IU
Vitamin C: 8mg
Folate: 5mcg

TIPS:

Always wash apples. Supermarket apples are often waxed, which can seal in pesticide residues that are on the skin. Peeling apples will remove the film but also a lot of fiber. To prevent browning once an apple is sliced, sprinkle some lemon juice on cut surfaces.

APRICOTS

For such diminutive, delicate fruit, apricots are a surprisingly robust source of fiber, beta-carotene, iron, and potassium.

BENEFITS:

Apricots are abundant in soluble fiber, which helps lower blood cholesterol levels. But the real heart-related news about apricots is that they're brimming with vitamin A (beta-carotene), an important antioxidant that's linked to the prevention of certain cancers, cataracts, and heart disease. And the potassium they provide helps maintain normal blood pressure. Be aware that sugar is often added during commercial canning, and the high heat used in the process destroys some nutrients. The drying process concentrates the nutrients, including the carbohydrates, so a half-cup serving of dried apricots has three times the calories of a single serving of fresh.

NUTRIENTS PER SERVING:

Apricot, 1 raw
Calories: 17
Protein: <1g
Total fat: 0g
Saturated fat: 0g
Cholesterol: 0g
Carbohydrate: 4g
Dietary fiber: 0.5g
Sodium: 0mg
Calcium: 5mg
Potassium: 90mg
Vitamin A: 764 IU
Folate: 0mcg

HOW TO SELECT AND STORE:

Fresh apricots are fragile and must be handled with care. Look for plump, golden-orange apricots that are fairly firm. You may need to ripen the fruit for a day or two at room temperature before you can enjoy them. Don't pile them up, as the pressure will cause them to bruise as they ripen. Once ripe, store them in the refrigerator. Canned and dried apricots offer delicious alternatives to fresh.

TIPS:

Be gentle when washing fresh apricots. To reap the most health benefits, eat the skins. If you use canned apricots, rinse them before eating to wash away the sugar-rich syrup. Fresh apricots make a great snack, and they can be sliced and put on salads, oatmeal, or yogurt.

APRICOT BISCOTTI

3 cups all-purpose flour

1½ teaspoons baking soda

½ teaspoon salt

⅔ cup sugar

3 eggs

1 teaspoon vanilla

½ cup chopped dried apricots

⅓ cup sliced almonds, chopped

1 tablespoon reduced-fat (2%) milk

1. Preheat oven to 350°F. Lightly coat cookie sheet with nonstick cooking spray; set aside.

2. Combine flour, baking soda, and salt in medium bowl; set aside.

3. Beat sugar, eggs, and vanilla in large bowl with electric mixer at medium speed until blended. Add flour mixture; beat until well blended.

4. Stir in apricots and almonds. Turn dough out onto lightly floured work surface. Knead 4 to 6 times. Shape dough into 20-inch log; place on prepared cookie sheet. Brush dough with milk.

5. Bake 30 minutes or until firm. Remove from oven; cool 10 minutes. Diagonally slice into 30 biscotti. Place slices on cookie sheet; bake 10 minutes. Turn and bake an additional 10 minutes. Cool on wire racks. Store in airtight container.

Makes 30 cookies

ARTICHOKES

Many would-be artichoke lovers shy away from this delicate, buttery-flavored vegetable because they don't know how to handle it. But artichokes require little prep work. What takes time is eating them!

BENEFITS:

The artichoke is a low-calorie vegetable that's rich in insoluble fiber, making it a nutritious choice for people with diabetes—as long as it's not dunked in a traditional, fat- and calorie-heavy dipping sauce, such as hollandaise or butter. Compared to the artichoke heart, the meaty leaves contain more nutrients, including potassium and folate.

HOW TO SELECT AND STORE:

Globe artichokes are commonly available in the produce department. Baby artichokes come from a side thistle of the plant. Artichoke hearts are the meaty base and are available canned. They can be used instead of fresh in many dishes including pasta medleys and salads. Look for fresh artichokes with a soft green color and tightly packed, closed leaves. Store artichokes in a plastic bag in the refrigerator; add a few drops of water to prevent them from drying out. Although best if used within a few days, they'll keep for a week or two if stored properly.

NUTRIENTS PER SERVING:

Artichoke, 1 medium cooked
Calories: 64
Protein: 3g
Total fat: 0g
Saturated fat: 0g
Cholesterol: 0g
Carbohydrate: 14g
Dietary fiber: 10g
Sodium: 70mg
Potassium: 340mg
Calcium: 25mg
Iron: 0.7mg
Vitamin A: 16 IU
Vitamin C: 9mg
Folate: 107mcg

TIPS:

Wash artichokes under running water. Pull off outer, lower leaves and trim the sharp tips. Boil in a saucepan for 20 to 40 minutes or steam for 25 to 40 minutes or until a center petal pulls out easily. Artichokes can be served hot or cold. Enjoy the rich flavor with lemon juice and a dash of olive oil.

AVOCADO

Often mistaken for a vegetable, this rich, smooth-textured fruit is most widely recognized when served as guacamole. Its buttery flavor is a good complement in vegetable, meat, salad, and pasta dishes.

BENEFITS:

Avocadoes frequently show up on lists of "super foods" for their numerous health benefits. Avocados are rich in monounsaturated fat, a type of fat recommended for a diabetic diet because it can lower LDL (bad) cholesterol, especially when it replaces saturated fat. Still, even the good kind of fat found in avocados is high in calories, so portion control is important. Avocados also contain lutein, which helps maintain healthy eyes and skin. They also contain healthy amounts of fiber, potassium, and vitamins C, K, and B_6.

NUTRIENTS PER SERVING:

Avocado, ½ fresh
Calories: 161
Protein: 2g
Total fat: 15g
Saturated fat: 2g
Cholesterol: 0g
Carbohydrate: 9g
Dietary fiber: 6.5g
Sodium: 5mg
Potassium: 485mg
Calcium: 12mg
Iron: 0.5mg
Vitamin A: 147 IU
Vitamin C: 10mg
Folate: 81mcg

HOW TO SELECT AND STORE:

The two most common varieties of avocados are the pebbly textured, dark-colored Haas and the green Fuerte, with its thin, smooth skin. Ripe avocados yield to gentle pressure and should be unblemished and heavy for their size. If you don't plan to use them right away, make sure you choose avocados that are firm. To speed up ripening, place avocados in a brown bag on the counter. Once ripened, they can be stored in the refrigerator for several days.

TIPS:

Avocados should be served raw, because they have a bitter taste when cooked. Avocado flesh browns rapidly when cut and exposed to air. Adding the avocado to a dish at the last moment can help minimize this, as can tossing cut avocado with a little lemon or lime juice.

BARLEY

This flavorful Middle Eastern grain helps curb appetite due to its fiber. Fiber's bulking ability makes it a great addition to any diet because it fills you up, reducing the likelihood you'll overindulge in a meal.

BENEFITS:

Even though barley is mostly carbohydrate, its soluble fiber helps slow digestion and regulate blood sugar. It's also rich in insoluble fiber, which adds bulk and speeds up the passing of intestinal contents through the body, possibly reducing colorectal cancer risk. Barley also provides B vitamins, iron, and magnesium.

HOW TO SELECT AND STORE:

Hulled, or whole grain, barley has had only its outer husk removed, so it's the most nutritious, with twice the fiber, vitamins, and minerals of pearl (polished) barley. Scotch barley is husked and coarsely ground and more nutritious than pearl. The most common form, pearl barley, has had its bran removed, so it's lowest in fiber, vitamins, and minerals, but still quite nutritious. It cooks quicker than hulled or Scotch. Quick barley is pearl barley that's pre-steamed to cook even faster. Store barley in an airtight container in a cool, dark place.

TIPS:

To cook, add 1 cup pearl barley to 2 cups boiling water or 1 cup hulled barley to 3 cups boiling water. Simmer, covered, until all water is absorbed, 10 to 15 minutes for quick barley, 45 to 55 minutes for pearl, and 60 to 90 minutes for hulled. You can soak hulled barley overnight to reduce cooking time. Barley is an excellent thickener for soups and stews.

NUTRIENTS PER SERVING:

Barley (pearl), ½ cup cooked
Calories: 97
Protein: 2g
Total fat: 0g
Saturated fat: 0g
Cholesterol: 0g
Carbohydrate: 22g
Dietary fiber: 3g
Sodium: 0mg
Potassium: 73mg
Calcium: 9mg
Iron: 1mg
Vitamin A: 5 IU
Folate: 13mcg

BEEF TENDERLOIN

Surprise! There's no need to ban beef from your diet. Considered one of the 29 lean cuts of beef, beef tenderloin contains only 8 grams of fat per 3-ounce serving—that's less than a skinless chicken thigh!

BENEFITS:

Lean beef provides quality protein and essential vitamins and minerals. Its easily absorbed iron is especially valuable, since a shortage of this mineral is a common nutritional deficiency. Half the fat in beef is heart-healthy monounsaturated fat. And a third of beef's saturated fat is a unique type shown to have a neutral effect on blood cholesterol. Short- and long-term studies indicate lean beef can fit in diets for lowering blood cholesterol.

HOW TO SELECT AND STORE:

Choose beef with a bright cherry-red or purplish color without any gray or brown blotches. Purchase tightly sealed packages and refrigerate or freeze beef as soon as possible. Use refrigerated beef within four days after purchase. To keep beef tenderloin lean, trim all fat from the exterior. To find other lean beef cuts, look for "loin" or "round" in the name.

NUTRIENTS PER SERVING:

Beef tenderloin, trimmed of all fat, 3 ounces roasted

Calories: 174
Protein: 23g
Total fat: 8g
Saturated fat: 8g
Cholesterol: 72g
Carbohydrate: 0g
Dietary fiber: 0g
Sodium: 50mg
Potassium: 280mg
Iron: 1.4mg
Zinc: 4.2mg
Phosphorus: 184mg
Vitamin B$_6$: 0.5mg
Vitamin B$_{12}$: 1.2mcg

TIPS:

Tender beef cuts, like tenderloin, are best prepared with a dry-heat cooking method, such as roasting, grilling, broiling, or stir-frying. These methods require little or no added fat. When using a marinade, tender cuts need only 15 minutes to 2 hours to add flavor. A seasoning rub is another great way to add flavor to the surface of beef. Cook to an internal temperature of at least 145°F for medium rare.

BELL PEPPERS

Bell peppers, or sweet peppers, come in a spectrum of hues. They're perfect for adding color, flavor, and crunch to a host of low-calorie dishes.

BENEFITS:

All bell peppers are rich in vitamins A and C, but red peppers contain the highest amounts. Bell peppers actually contain more vitamin C by weight than any of the citrus fruits. Vitamins A and C are antioxidants that help prevent cell damage, inflammation, cancer, and diseases related to aging, as well as support immune function. Bell peppers also contain lutein, an antioxidant linked to reduced risk of macular degeneration. They additionally provide a decent dose of fiber.

HOW TO SELECT AND STORE:

Green peppers are simply red, orange, or yellow peppers that have yet to ripen. As they ripen, they get sweeter and turn various shades until they reach their mature color. Once ripe, they are more perishable. Regardless of age, bell peppers should have a glossy sheen and no shriveling, cracks, or soft spots. Select those that are heavy for their size. Store peppers in a plastic bag in your refrigerator's crisper drawer. Green bell peppers stay firm for a week; other colors go soft in three or four days.

TIPS:

Bell pepper slices are delicious raw—in a salad, with a low-fat dip, or alone. They develop a stronger flavor when cooked. They can be bitter when overcooked. Add bell peppers to stir-fries and pasta dishes.

NUTRIENTS PER SERVING:

Bell peppers (red), ½ cup raw, sliced
Calories: 14
Protein: 1g
Total fat: 0g
Saturated fat: 0g
Cholesterol: 0g
Carbohydrate: 3g
Dietary fiber: 1g
Sodium: 0mg
Potassium: 97mg
Calcium: 3mg
Iron: 0.2mg
Vitamin A: 1,440 IU
Vitamin C: 59mg
Folate: 21mcg

BLACK BEANS

What food is high in protein, has virtually no fat, and contains more fiber than most whole grains? Beans! Dried beans are the seeds of plants called legumes, and they're a valuable, versatile food.

BENEFITS:

Like other legumes, black beans are packed with filling fiber, vitamins, and minerals. The soluble fiber in black beans slows digestion and blunts the rise of blood sugar after meals.

The American Diabetes Association considers beans a "super food" since just a ½ cup gives you about a third your daily requirement of fiber and as much protein as an ounce of meat, without the saturated fat. Eating a mere 3 cups of beans a week can help reduce the risk of heart disease and certain cancers.

HOW TO SELECT AND STORE:

Both dried and canned black beans are available all year long. Dried black beans stored in an airtight container will last a year or more. Once cooked, they'll keep in the refrigerator for about four days, or in the freezer for up to six months.

NUTRIENTS PER SERVING:

Black beans, ½ cup cooked (no salt or fat added)
Calories: 99
Protein: 6g
Total fat: 0g
Saturated fat: 0g
Cholesterol: 0mg
Carbohydrate: 18g
Dietary fiber: 4g
Sodium: 4mg
Folate: 65mcg
Potassium: 322mg
Iron: 1mg
Magnesium: 40mg
Copper: 176mcg

TIPS:

Many cultures have perfected the art of combining black beans with grains to provide a complete meal rich in protein. Black beans make a tasty addition to soups and chilis. Try Mexican dishes with black beans in place of traditional refried beans. Black beans, corn, and fresh cilantro can perk up any salsa. If using canned beans, be sure to drain and rinse the beans to reduce sodium.

BLACK-EYED PEAS

Tradition suggests eating black-eyed peas on New Year's Day will bring good fortune in the coming year. But this legendary legume brings more than good luck.

BENEFITS:

Black-eyed peas, also called cowpeas, bring a winning combination of fiber and protein to a diabetic diet. The fiber is mostly soluble, so it helps lower cholesterol and regulates blood sugar. Not only are black-eyed peas very low in fat, they have fewer calories and carbohydrates than other legumes. They provide calcium, iron, potassium, magnesium, and folate, too.

HOW TO SELECT AND STORE:

Store fresh black-eyed peas in a plastic bag in your refrigerator's vegetable drawer and use them within a week. If fresh aren't available, dry, canned, and frozen are nutritious alternatives. If you opt for dry black-eyed peas, look for ones that have some shine. If you're using canned, choose a variety with no added salt, or drain and rinse the beans under cool water after opening.

TIPS:

Black-eyed peas can be used in soups or casseroles or served as a side dish. They are the main ingredient in the traditional New Year's Hoppin' John, which includes bacon or other high-fat ingredients, so try and use lower-fat alternatives when serving up this savory dish. Dried black-eyed peas should be soaked overnight before cooking. Canned varieties may be too soft for some recipes.

NUTRIENTS PER SERVING:

Black-eyed peas, ½ cup cooked
Calories: 80
Protein: 3g
Total fat: 0g
Saturated fat: 0g
Cholesterol: 0g
Carbohydrate: 17g
Dietary fiber: 4g
Sodium: 0mg
Potassium: 345mg
Calcium: 106mg
Iron: 0.9mg
Vitamin A: 653 IU
Vitamin C: 2mg
Folate: 105mcg

BLACKBERRIES

Blackberries are a wonder food. When fully ripe, they are sweet and juicy, yet they are low in calories and high in fiber. They are great for baking or just eating out of hand.

BENEFITS:

Fresh blackberries are an excellent source of vitamin C. Even more notable is their fiber; a handful has more fiber than a serving of some whole grain cereals. They are packed with soluble fiber, which slows absorption of sugar and helps steady blood sugar levels. Their nearly black appearance comes from high levels of anthocyanins and ellagic acid, two phytonutrients with numerous health benefits, including helping to prevent heart disease and cancer and combating aging.

HOW TO SELECT AND STORE:

Look for berries that are glossy, deep-colored, plump, well rounded, and firm. The darker the berries, the riper and sweeter they are.

Refrigerate blackberries, but don't wash them until you're ready to eat them, or they can get moldy. They are best if used within a day or two. To enjoy fresh blackberries year-round, place the washed and dried berries in a single layer on a cookie sheet in the freezer; once frozen, place them in an airtight container and thaw as needed.

TIPS:

Wash blackberries gently under running water, drain well, and remove stems and berries that are too soft. Do not over-handle them, or their cells will break open and they will lose juice and nutrients. Enjoy fresh blackberries alone, over cereal or yogurt, or with a refreshing scoop of sorbet.

NUTRIENTS PER SERVING:

Blackberries, ½ cup raw
Calories: 31
Protein: 1g
Total fat: 0g
Saturated fat: 0g
Cholesterol: 0g
Carbohydrate: 7g
Dietary fiber: 4g
Sodium: 0mg
Potassium: 120mg
Calcium: 21mg
Iron: 0.5mg
Vitamin A: 154 IU
Vitamin C: 15mg
Folate: 18mcg

BLUEBERRIES

Blueberries are antioxidant superstars, ranking second among top antioxidant-rich foods. These flavorful berries are a true health bargain.

BENEFITS:

Besides being packed with antioxidants, blueberries are a good source of fiber and provide vitamin C and iron. Recent research suggests that eating blueberries as part of a healthy diet may help reduce several key risk factors for cardiovascular disease and diabetes, such as accumulation of belly fat, high blood cholesterol, and high blood sugar. Antioxidants in blueberries may also protect your eyes and brain cells and help reverse age-related memory loss.

HOW TO SELECT AND STORE:

Blueberries are best when they are in season, from May through October. Choose blueberries that are firm, uniform in size, and indigo blue with a silvery frost. Discard shriveled or moldy berries. Don't wash them until you're ready to use them. Store in a moisture-proof container in the refrigerator for up to five days. Freeze washed and dried blueberries in a single layer on a cookie sheet, and place in a sealed container once frozen.

NUTRIENTS PER SERVING:
Blueberries, ½ cup raw
Calories: 42
Protein: 1g
Total fat: 0g
Saturated fat: 0g
Cholesterol: 0g
Carbohydrate: 11g
Dietary fiber: 2g
Sodium: 0mg
Potassium: 60mg
Calcium: 4mg
Iron: 0.2mg
Vitamin A: 401 IU
Vitamin C: 7mg
Folate: 4mcg

TIPS:

Enjoy blueberries on cereal, in yogurt or salads, with a splash of cream, or simply out of hand. Blueberry jam is a nutritious low-fat spread. Frozen blueberries make a refreshing snack and are a great addition to smoothies. Once frozen, blueberries are best used in baking, as they become mushy once thawed. Blueberries are easy to bake into muffins, pancakes, quick breads, pies, cobblers, and fruit crisps.

BLUEBERRY CUSTARD SUPREME

½ cup fresh blueberries

2 tablespoons all-purpose flour

1½ tablespoons granulated sugar

⅛ teaspoon salt

¼ teaspoon ground cardamom

¼ cup cholesterol-free egg substitute

1 teaspoon grated lemon peel

½ teaspoon vanilla

¾ cup reduced-fat (2%) milk

1 teaspoon powdered sugar

1. Preheat oven to 350°F. Spray 1-quart soufflé or casserole dish with nonstick cooking spray. Distribute blueberries over bottom of prepared dish.

2. Whisk flour, granulated sugar, salt, and cardamom in small bowl. Add egg substitute, lemon peel, and vanilla; whisk until smooth and well blended. Whisk in milk. Pour over blueberries.

3. Bake 30 minutes or until puffed, lightly browned and center is set. Cool on wire rack. Serve warm or at room temperature. Sprinkle with powdered sugar just before serving.

Makes 2 servings

NUTRIENTS PER SERVING:

Calories: 155
Calories from fat: 11%
Total fat: 2g
Saturated fat: 1g
Protein: 7g
Carbohydrate: 27g
Cholesterol: 7mg
Sodium: 249mg
Dietary fiber: 1g
Dietary exchanges:
½ Fruit, 1 Starch, ½ Milk

BROCCOLI

Whether eaten raw or cooked, you are truly getting a powerhouse of nutrients when you incorporate this cruciferous vegetable into your diet. Broccoli complements other flavors and textures.

BENEFITS:

Broccoli's noteworthy nutrients include vitamin C, vitamin A (mostly as the antioxidant beta-carotene), folate, calcium, and fiber. It's a great nutritional bargain for a diabetes meal plan because in addition to being low in fat and calories, it's one of the vegetables lowest in sugars and carbohydrates. Broccoli is rich in an array of phytonutrients that serve as powerful cancer fighters, helping to inhibit tumor growth and boost the action of protective enzymes.

HOW TO SELECT AND STORE:

Look for broccoli that's dark green or even purplish-green, but avoid yellow. Florets should be compact and of even color, leaves should not be wilted, and stalks should not be fat and woody. The greener it is, the more beta-carotene it has. Store unwashed broccoli in a plastic bag in the refrigerator's crisper drawer. Use within a few days.

TIPS:

Wash broccoli just before using. Steaming is the best way to retain nutrients. Steam only until crisp-tender, about five minutes. Broccoli florets can boost the texture, flavor, and color of any stir-fry dish. Raw broccoli tossed into salads boosts the nutrition of a midday meal. For a healthier side dish, skip the cheese sauce. Instead, add a squeeze of lemon and a dusting of cracked pepper or a drizzle of olive oil.

NUTRIENTS PER SERVING:

Broccoli, ½ cup cooked
Calories: 27
Protein: 2g
Total fat: 0g
Saturated fat: 0g
Cholesterol: 0g
Carbohydrate: 6g
Dietary fiber: 3g
Sodium: 32mg
Potassium: 229mg
Calcium: 31mg
Iron: 0.5mg
Vitamin A: 1,207 IU
Vitamin C: 51mg
Folate: 84mcg

BROCCOLI RABE

The Italians have been eating broccoli rabe for years, but it has only recently become mainstream due to its nutritional benefits and savory qualities. This vegetable, closely related to turnips and cabbage (not broccoli), is also known as broccoli raab or rapini.

BENEFITS:

Like its cruciferous-vegetable relatives, broccoli rabe supplies a hefty dose of health-promoting nutrients. It's great for diabetics as it is low in calories, sugars, and carbohydrates. Just a ½ cup provides more than 10 percent of the recommended daily amounts of fiber, potassium, folate, and calcium, and more than 50 percent of the daily recommendations for vitamins A and C. Plus, it's packed with powerful, cancer-fighting phytonutrients.

HOW TO SELECT AND STORE:

Broccoli rabe can be found from fall to spring in specialty produce sections.

NUTRIENTS PER SERVING:

Broccoli rabe, ½ cup cooked
Calories: 38
Protein: 4g
Total fat: 0.5g
Saturated fat: 0g
Cholesterol: 0g
Carbohydrate: 4g
Dietary fiber: 3g
Sodium: 64mg
Calcium: 136mg
Potassium: 390mg
Iron: 1.5mg
Vitamin A: 5,213 IU
Vitamin C: 43mg
Folate: 82mcg

Look for broccoli rabe that is bright green with firm, crisp leaves, broccoli-like buds, and thin stalks, free of yellowing and spotting. Wrap loosely in a plastic bag and refrigerate for up to five days. After cooking, refrigerate leftovers in a sealed container for up to two days.

TIPS:

If you find the flavor too strong, blanch it in boiling water for 30 to 60 seconds before cooking it. Because it's tough, broccoli rabe is usually steamed or sautéed. Remove an inch from each stem and peel the lower half of thick stems to reduce toughness. Broccoli rabe can easily complement heavy, spiced entrées. Or sauté it in olive oil with red pepper flakes and minced garlic and serve alone.

BROWN RICE

Many people think this comfort food has no place in a diabetic diet. But brown rice is actually a pantry staple for those with diabetes. Not only is it nutritionally superior to white rice, it has a nuttier flavor and chewier texture from its natural bran coating.

BENEFITS:

Brown rice is considered a whole grain, so it's an excellent source of complex carbohydrates, especially fiber. In fact, it has three times the fiber of the ever-so-popular white rice. Brown rice naturally contains more magnesium, phosphorus, manganese, and selenium than white. Research has shown that brown rice helps regulate glucose metabolism in people with diabetes, likely due to its high fiber and mineral content.

HOW TO SELECT AND STORE:

Brown rice is more perishable than white rice and keeps about six months or longer if refrigerated. It is available in several forms: regular brown rice in long and short grain; quick brown rice, which has been partially cooked and dehydrated; and instant brown rice, which has been fully cooked and dehydrated. The main difference among the varieties is cooking time.

TIPS:

Long grain brown rice takes about 30 minutes to cook; short grain brown rice takes about 40 minutes. Instant and quick-cooking varieties cook in 10 to 15 minutes. For tasty, satisfying, and nutrient-rich meals, serve brown rice with stir-fries with plenty of vegetables and a little lean meat or tofu. Or try a cool rice salad with peas, red peppers, and a warm low-fat vinaigrette dressing.

NUTRIENTS PER SERVING:

Brown rice (long grain), ½ cup cooked
Calories: 108
Protein: 3g
Total fat: 1g
Saturated fat: 0g
Cholesterol: 0g
Carbohydrate: 22g
Dietary fiber: 2g
Sodium: 5mg
Potassium: 40mg
Iron: 0.4mg
Magnesium: 42mg
Phosphorus: 81mg
Manganese: 0.9mg
Selenium: 9.6mcg

BUCKWHEAT

Despite its name, buckwheat is not a type of wheat nor is it a grain; it's the seed from an herb. Buckwheat is commonly found hulled and crushed as groats, roasted groats, or kasha.

BENEFITS:

Buckwheat contains more protein than grains do, and its protein is more nutritionally complete, which makes it a particularly good base for meatless meals. It's a healthy source of fiber, which helps fill you up and even out your blood sugar levels. Additionally, studies have shown that a phytochemical found in buckwheat may actually be capable of lowering blood sugar.

HOW TO SELECT AND STORE:

You can buy groats whole, cracked into coarse, medium, or fine grinds, or roasted as kasha. Very finely cracked unroasted groats, or buckwheat grits, are sold as a hot cereal. Buckwheat flour is available in light and dark, depending on the amount of hull. Darker versions have more fiber and a stronger flavor. Keep buckwheat in a well-sealed container in the refrigerator or freezer. At room temperature, it is susceptible to turning rancid.

NUTRIENTS PER SERVING:

Buckwheat (kasha), ½ cup cooked

Calories: 77
Protein: 3g
Total fat: 0.5g
Saturated fat: 0g
Cholesterol: 0g
Carbohydrate: 17g
Dietary fiber: 2g
Sodium: 0mg
Potassium: 70mg
Calcium: 6mg
Iron: 0.7mg
Magnesium: 43mg
Folate: 12mcg

TIPS:

Buckwheat has an intense, nutty flavor. Cook groats or kasha like rice, following package instructions. You can substitute buckwheat groats or kasha in most recipes calling for rice or other whole grains. Buckwheat can be found as a traditional kasha soup in Jewish delis and also as soba noodles in popular Japanese dishes. Buckwheat is not recommended for baking.

BULGUR

This tasty Middle Eastern staple consists of wheat kernels that have been steamed, dried, and crushed. It's an inexpensive, low-fat source of protein, making it a wonderfully nutritious and economical addition to any meal plan.

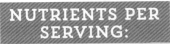
Bulgur, ½ cup cooked
Calories: 76
Protein: 3g
Total fat: 0g
Saturated fat: 0g
Cholesterol: 0mg
Carbohydrate: 17g
Dietary fiber: 4g
Sodium: 5mg
Potassium: 60mg
Calcium: 9mg
Iron: 0.9mg
Folate: 16mcg

BENEFITS:

Bulgur makes an ideal foundation for diabetes-wise meal plans. It doesn't lose many nutrients during its minimal processing, remaining high in protein and minerals. Its low-fat, low-calorie profile and generous dose of fiber make it a superstar ingredient. Bulgur makes an excellent stand-in for fatty, calorie-laden protein sources, including meats, making it an especially helpful menu addition for people with diabetes who need to lose weight.

HOW TO SELECT AND STORE:

Bulgur is available in three grinds—coarse, medium, and fine. Coarse bulgur is used to make pilaf or stuffing. Medium-grind bulgur is used in cereals. The finest grind of bulgur is used in the popular Middle Eastern cold salad called tabbouleh. Store bulgur in a screw-top glass jar in the refrigerator. It will keep for months.

TIPS:

Because bulgur is already partially cooked, little time is needed for preparation. Simply combine ½ cup of bulgur with 1 cup of liquid and simmer for 15 minutes; let stand for 10 minutes and fluff with a fork. Bulgur triples in volume. If you like your bulgur chewier, let it sit longer to absorb more water. Bulgur can be used in place of rice in most recipes. Bulgur lends its nutty flavor to whatever it is combined with, allowing you to use it in a variety of dishes.

BUTTERNUT SQUASH

Sweet and buttery tasting, this satisfying and fiber-rich winter squash makes an excellent addition to a diabetic meal plan. Its tough shell allows for longer storage so it can be enjoyed into the winter.

BENEFITS:

Beta-carotene, the antioxidant form of vitamin A, is what gives butternut squash its deep orange-yellow color. This essential vitamin helps maintain eye health and promote healthy skin—both of which are of special concern to people with diabetes, who are at increased risk of certain eye diseases and skin ulcers. Plus, the fiber in butternut squash provides a feeling of fullness and slows the rise in blood sugar levels.

HOW TO SELECT AND STORE:

Butternut squash is available year-round; its peak season is from early fall through winter. It has a bulbous end and a smooth outer shell that ranges from yellow to camel-colored. Choose squash that is firm and free of bruises, punctures, or cuts. Uncooked, it does not need refrigeration and can be stored in a cool, dark place for several weeks.

NUTRIENTS PER SERVING:

Butternut squash, ½ cup cooked
Calories: 41
Protein: 1g
Total fat: 0g
Saturated fat: 0g
Cholesterol: 0mg
Carbohydrate: 11g
Dietary fiber: 3.5g
Sodium: 0mg
Potassium: 290mg
Calcium: 42mg
Iron: 0.6mg
Vitamin A: 11,434 IU
Vitamin C: 16mg
Folate: 19mcg

TIPS:

The simplest way to prepare butternut squash is to cut it in half and bake or microwave. To help soften for easier cutting, microwave the squash for 3 to 5 minutes. Cut it lengthwise, scoop out the seeds, and proceed with cooking or peeling. Cube peeled squash and add it to soups or stews, or simply mash and season with cinnamon or go savory with garlic and Parmesan cheese.

CANTALOUPE

It's hard to say no to this melon with its soft, sweet, juicy flesh, and superb taste. Fortunately, there's no need to! Cantaloupe is the perfect substitute for sugary, processed snacks and desserts in a diabetic diet.

BENEFITS:

Cantaloupe is a good source of potassium, an essential nutrient that may help lower high blood pressure, regulate heartbeat, and prevent strokes and heart disease. But this succulent melon's potential to protect against heart and blood-vessel diseases doesn't stop there. Cantaloupe is also rich in beta-carotene, vitamin C, and phytonutrients, a powerful trio that helps prevent cardiovascular disease, cancer, and infection. Because it's mostly water, cantaloupe is low in calories, yet its fiber content and sweet taste make it satisfying.

NUTRIENTS PER SERVING:

Cantaloupe, ½ cup raw
Calories: 27
Protein: 1g
Total fat: 0g
Saturated fat: 0g
Cholesterol: 0mg
Carbohydrate: 7g
Dietary fiber: 1g
Sodium: 10mg
Potassium: 210mg
Calcium: 7mg
Iron: 0.2mg
Vitamin A: 2,706 IU
Vitamin C: 29mg
Folate: 17mcg

HOW TO SELECT AND STORE:

Look for evenly shaped cantaloupes without bruises, cracks, or soft spots. Select ones that are heavy for their size. Ripe cantaloupes have a mildly sweet fragrance. Avoid cantaloupe that smells sickeningly sweet, or has mold where the stem used to be. Cantaloupes continue to ripen off the vine, so if you buy it ripe, eat it as soon as possible.

TIPS:

Enjoy cantaloupe slightly chilled or at room temperature for the most flavor. Chilled melon soup is refreshing in hot weather. And the natural cavity left in a cantaloupe after removing the seeds is a perfect place for fillers like nonfat yogurt or fruit salad. Squeeze a little lemon or lime juice onto cut melon for extra flavor.

CARROTS

Because carrots are sweeter than many other vegetables, many think of them as being higher in sugar. But sweeter doesn't always mean higher in carbohydrates. Sweet, crunchy carrots are a delicious and nutritious addition to any diet.

BENEFITS:

Carrots' substantial fiber and low carbohydrate content combined with their high vitamin A content make these popular vegetables a super food. Carrots are great for anyone watching what they eat. Carrots' soluble fiber provides a feeling of fullness without adding calories. The soluble fiber also helps lower blood cholesterol levels, which are often elevated in people with diabetes. When it comes to beta-carotene, carrots have few rivals. A mere ½ cup serving packs a huge amount of this antioxidant form of vitamin A. Beta-carotene helps defend the body's cells from damage, including cells in the heart, blood vessels, and eyes, which are more vulnerable due to diabetes.

NUTRIENTS PER SERVING:

Carrots, ½ cup raw
Calories: 25
Protein: 1g
Total fat: 0g
Saturated fat: 0g
Cholesterol: 0mg
Carbohydrate: 6g
Dietary fiber: 2g
Sodium: 40mg
Potassium: 195mg
Calcium: 20mg
Iron: 0.2mg
Vitamin A: 10,191 IU
Vitamin C: 4mg
Folate: 12mcg

HOW TO SELECT AND STORE:

Look for firm carrots with bright orange color and smooth skin. Avoid carrots if they are limp or black near the tops. Choose medium-sized ones that taper at the ends. Thicker carrots may be tough. Baby-cut carrots are sweet and convenient. All carrots will keep for a few weeks.

TIPS:

Wash and scrub whole carrots to remove soil contaminants. To remove pesticides, peel the outer layer and cut off ¼ inch off the fat end. Carrots are a great raw snack, but their true sweet flavor shines when cooked. Very little nutritional value is lost in cooking.

CARROT CAKE

2 cups cake flour
2 teaspoons ground cinnamon
1 teaspoon baking powder
1 teaspoon baking soda
1 teaspoon salt
¾ cup sugar substitute
¾ cup packed brown sugar
¼ cup vegetable oil
1 cup cholesterol-free egg substitute

¾ cup reduced-fat sour cream, divided
3 cups grated carrots
4 ounces fat-free cream cheese, softened
1 tablespoon fat-free (skim) milk
1 teaspoon vanilla
½ cup powdered sugar

1. Preheat oven to 350°F. Spray 12-cup bundt pan with nonstick cooking spray.

NUTRIENTS PER SERVING:

Carrot cake, 1 slice
Calories: 176
Calories from fat: 26%
Protein: 5g
Total fat: 5g
Saturated fat: 1g
Cholesterol: 5mg
Carbohydrate: 28g
Fiber: 1g
Sodium: 357mg
Dietary exchanges:
2 Starch, ½ Fat

2. Combine flour, cinnamon, baking powder, baking soda, and salt in medium bowl. Beat sugar substitute, brown sugar, and oil in large bowl with electric mixer at medium speed. Beat in egg substitute and ½ cup of the sour cream. Slowly add flour mixture, beating at low speed just until blended. Stir in carrots. Pour batter into prepared pan.

3. Bake 50 minutes or until toothpick inserted near center comes out clean. Let stand 5 minutes. Invert cake onto wire rack; cool completely.

4. Whisk cream cheese, remaining ¼ cup sour cream, milk, and vanilla in small bowl until smooth. Whisk in powdered sugar. If glaze is too thick, add water, 1 teaspoon at a time, until desired consistency. Spoon glaze evenly over cake. Cut into 16 slices.

Makes 16 servings

CASHEWS

This delicately flavored nut is a wise nut choice for people with diabetes. Researchers are studying the potential role of cashew-nut extract in the treatment of the disease.

BENEFITS:

Cashews have long been used to treat high blood sugar, and recent research suggests an extract of the nut may improve the ability to respond to insulin. Cashews are also rich in magnesium, a mineral that has been associated with insulin resistance when it is lacking in the diet, as well as high blood pressure and other traits that increase the risk of heart disease, stroke, and diabetes. Cashews are lower in fat than many other popular nuts and contain little saturated fat. The fat they do contain is primarily monounsaturated oleic acid, which is considered heart healthy. Like other nuts, cashews provide protein and fiber, making them filling and satisfying.

NUTRIENTS PER SERVING:

Cashews, 1 ounce dry roasted without salt
Calories: 163
Protein: 4g
Total fat: 13g
Saturated fat: 2.5g
Cholesterol: 0mg
Carbohydrate: 9g
Dietary fiber: 1g
Sodium: 5mg
Potassium: 160mg
Iron: 1.7mg
Vitamin E: 0.3mg
Magnesium: 74mg
Folate: 20mcg

HOW TO SELECT AND STORE:

Cashews are available oil roasted and salted, but are most nutritious in their dry roasted and unsalted form. Because of their fat content, they should be stored in an airtight container, in the refrigerator, to prevent rancidity. Always check the "sell by" date on packages of cashews to be sure they are fresh.

TIPS:

Cashews make wonderful nut butter and a tasty addition to salads and stir-fry dishes. As with most nuts, roasting cashews intensifies their flavor so you can use less in recipes. Enjoy cashews as a snack, but be sure to watch your portions.

CHEESE

Any way you slice it, cheese adds creaminess and a rich flavor to foods. Although high in fat, a little cheese goes a long way. A sprinkling of Parmesan cheese over a vegetable dish or a snack of fruit accompanied by a bit of Cheddar are indulgences that can also make nutritional sense.

BENEFITS:

Cheese is low in carbohydrates and has very little effect on blood sugar levels. Its protein makes it a long-lasting energy source, but because it can be high in fat, it's a food to enjoy in moderation. Cheese is a concentrated source of many of the nutrients found in milk, including calcium, protein, phosphorus, magnesium, potassium, vitamin A, riboflavin, and vitamin B_{12}.

HOW TO SELECT AND STORE:

There are more than 300 varieties of cheese, many available in various flavors and forms (sliced, cubed, shredded, spreadable, etc.). Choose reduced-fat or part-skim varieties for fewer calories and less fat. Purchase cheese by the "sell by" date and store it, tightly wrapped, in the refrigerator's cheese compartment for up to several weeks.

NUTRIENTS PER SERVING:

Cheese, 1 ounce reduced-fat provolone
Calories: 77
Protein: 7g
Total fat: 5g
Saturated fat: 3g
Cholesterol: 15mg
Carbohydrate: 1g
Dietary fiber: 0g
Sodium: 245mg
Potassium: 39mg
Calcium: 212mg
Iron: 0.2mg
Vitamin A: 149 IU
Phosphorus: 139mg
Vitamin B_{12}: 0.4mcg

TIPS:

Cheese can be eaten alone or added to other dishes. A little cheese pairs well with fruits, vegetables, and grains, making these foods even more nutritious and delicious. Full-flavored hard cheeses, such as Parmesan or Asiago, or aromatic sharp cheeses, such as sharp Cheddar or Gorgonzola, can be used in smaller amounts to add intense flavor to dishes without a ton of excess calories.

CHERRIES

Whether sweet or tart, dried or juiced, fresh, frozen, or canned, cherries pack a powerful nutritional punch. Sweet cherries make an ideal snack or dessert. Tart cherries offer important health benefits and work well in savory or sweet dishes.

BENEFITS:

Emerging evidence links cherries to important health benefits, from helping to ease the pain of arthritis and gout to reducing risk factors for heart disease, diabetes, and certain cancers. Compared to sweet cherries, tart (or sour) cherries are higher in vitamins and minerals, but both types provide disease-fighting antioxidants, including beta-carotene and vitamin C. Cherries supply potassium, which is essential for healthy blood pressure, and soluble fiber, which helps lower cholesterol and regulate blood sugar. Cherries also contain melatonin, which has been found to help regulate the body's natural sleep patterns and may even help prevent memory loss.

HOW TO SELECT AND STORE:

Most fresh cherries are available from May to August. Choose brightly colored, shiny, and plump cherries without blemishes. Store unwashed cherries in a plastic bag in the refrigerator. Cherries with stems tend to last longer, but are best when used within a few days. Dried cherries are available in sweet and sour varieties, but may contain added sugar.

TIPS:

Sweet cherries are best when eaten fresh, but they can also be cooked. For a sweet addition to salads, toss in dried or fresh sweet cherries. Most tart cherries are too sour to eat raw but make excellent sauces, pies, relishes, and preserves.

No-Bake Cherry Cake

1 (10-inch) prepared angel food cake

1½ cups fat-free (skim) milk

1 cup reduced-fat sour cream

1 package (4-serving size) vanilla fat-free sugar-free instant pudding and pie filling mix

1 can (21 ounces) cherry pie filling

NUTRIENTS PER SERVING:

Cherry cake, 1 piece (¹/₁₂ of cake)
Calories: 156
Calories from fat: 11%
Protein: 4g
Total fat: 2g
Saturated fat: 1g
Cholesterol: 7mg
Carbohydrate: 31g
Dietary fiber: 1g
Sodium: 326mg
Dietary exchanges:
1 Starch, 1 Milk, ½ Lean Meat

1. Tear cake into bite-size pieces; press into 11x7-inch baking dish.

2. Combine milk, sour cream, and pudding mix in medium bowl; beat with wire whisk or electric mixer at medium speed for 2 minutes or until thickened. Spread over cake in baking dish.

3. Spoon cherry pie filling evenly over top of cake. Chill; cut into 12 pieces to serve.

Makes 12 servings

CHICKEN BREAST

Chicken breast is a staple in any diet, as it is one of the leanest meats. It's a versatile source of high quality protein with significantly less saturated fat than other types of meats.

BENEFITS:

Of the edible parts of a chicken, the breast has the least fat. Removing the skin subtracts another 4 grams of fat (1 gram of it saturated, or "bad" fat) and roughly 60 calories. Chicken is also a good source of several B vitamins including vitamins B_6, B_{12}, and niacin, which are important for healthy immune function.

HOW TO SELECT AND STORE:

Chicken breasts are available in various forms. Whole breasts with the skin on are the most economical. For convenience, boneless, skinless chicken breasts are available; just be aware of pre-seasoned chicken breasts that are higher in sodium. Refrigerate raw chicken for up to two days, and cooked chicken up to three days. When freezing raw chicken, seal tightly in a plastic bag to prevent freezer burn. For best flavor and texture, use frozen chicken within two months.

TIPS:

To keep chicken breast lean, use a low-fat cooking method such as baking, roasting, grilling, broiling, or stewing. If not eating the skin, it makes little difference whether the skin is removed before or after cooking, but the meat is more moist and tender when cooked with the skin on. Cook chicken until the internal temperature is 165°F. Boneless chicken will cook faster than its bone-in counterpart.

NUTRIENTS PER SERVING:

Chicken breast, 3 ounces roasted, skinless

Calories: 140
Protein: 26g
Total fat: 3g
Saturated fat: 1g
Cholesterol: 72mg
Carbohydrate: 0g
Dietary fiber: 0g
Sodium: 60mg
Potassium: 22mg
Iron: 0.9mg
Vitamin B_6: 0.5mg
Vitamin B_{12}: 0.3mcg
Niacin: 12mcg

CHILI PEPPERS

Ranging from mild to very hot, chili peppers add tons of spice and flavor to many dishes. Emerging research suggests these little packages also pack a powerful punch for health, including helping to lower blood glucose levels.

BENEFITS:

Early research suggests capsaicin, the substance that gives chili peppers their characteristic bite, may help improve insulin's effectiveness in lowering blood sugar after meals. These findings could be valuable for both the prevention and treatment of type 2 diabetes. Chili peppers are also rich in beta-carotene and vitamin C, important antioxidants that fight heart disease, which is more common among people with diabetes.

NUTRIENTS PER SERVING:

Chili peppers (red), 2 tablespoons raw chopped

Calories: 8
Protein: 0g
Total fat: 0g
Saturated fat: 0g
Cholesterol: 0mg
Carbohydrate: 2g
Dietary fiber: <1g
Sodium: 0mg
Potassium: 60mg
Calcium: 3mg
Iron: 0.2mg
Vitamin A: 178 IU
Vitamin C: 27mg
Folate: 4mcg

HOW TO SELECT AND STORE:

Choose chili peppers based on the heat they provide. Mild to moderately hot peppers include Anaheim, ancho, and poblano peppers, while hotter varieties include cayenne, jalapeño, Serrano, and habanero. Fresh chili peppers should have a deep, vivid color with no shriveling. Store in the refrigerator's vegetable drawer. Chili peppers are available as chili pastes, hot sauces, flakes, and powders.

TIPS:

To cool the fire of hot peppers, cut away the inside white membrane and discard the seeds. Wash hands, utensils, and cutting board with soap and water after handling. Avoid touching your eyes. Chili peppers can be used in many types of dishes. Dried chili flakes are an easy way to add spice to pizzas, salads, soups, and chilis.

CINNAMON

Used for centuries as a culinary spice and for medicinal purposes, cinnamon is gaining attention as an aid for regulating blood sugar levels.

BENEFITS:

Several studies have shown improved insulin sensitivity and blood glucose control from taking as little as a ½ teaspoon of cinnamon per day. Cinnamon may also help lower blood cholesterol and triglyceride levels, which are often elevated in people with type 2 diabetes. Cinnamon contains more protective antioxidants than many other spices and foods do. You'll find as many antioxidants in 1 teaspoon of cinnamon as in a full cup of pomegranate juice or ½ cup of blueberries. Cinnamon is also a source of chromium, a mineral that enhances the action of insulin.

NUTRIENTS PER SERVING:

Cinnamon, 1 teaspoon ground
Calories: 6
Protein: 0g
Total fat: 0g
Saturated fat: 0g
Cholesterol: 0mg
Carbohydrate: 2g
Dietary fiber: 1g
Sodium: 0mg
Potassium: 11mg
Calcium: 26mg
Iron: 0.2mg
Vitamin A: 8 IU

HOW TO SELECT AND STORE:

Cinnamon is available ground or as sticks, or scrolls, of dried bark. Ground cinnamon has a stronger flavor than the sticks and can stay fresh for six months; the scrolls last longer. Both should be stored in a cool, dark, dry place.

TIPS:

Cinnamon adds a distinctive flavor to both sweet and savory dishes. It's often paired with apples and added to baked goods, but also adds a pungent flavor to Middle Eastern and Asian dishes. Cinnamon is an ingredient in curry powder. Be adventurous with cinnamon. Perk up drinks, such as coffee, tea, smoothies, or mulled wine, with ground cinnamon or sticks of cinnamon. Sprinkle cinnamon on cereal, ice cream, pudding, or yogurt. Add cinnamon to lamb or beef marinades.

CINNAMON-RAISIN BREAD PUDDING

1 can (12 ounces) evaporated skim milk

⅓ cup cholesterol free egg substitute

2 tablespoons sugar

3 teaspoons maple syrup, divided

¼ teaspoon vanilla

⅛ teaspoon ground cinnamon

4 slices cinnamon-raisin bread, torn into 1-inch pieces

NUTRIENTS PER SERVING:

Cinnamon-raisin bread pudding, ¼ total recipe
Calories: 192
Calories from fat: 6%
Protein: 11g
Total fat: 1g
Saturated fat: <1g
Cholesterol: 3mg
Carbohydrate: 34g
Dietary fiber: 0g
Sodium: 240mg
Calcium: 306mg
Dietary exchanges:
1½ Starch, 1 Milk

1. Preheat oven to 350°F. Spray 4 custard cups with nonstick cooking spray. Pour 2 cups water into 8x8-inch baking pan; set aside.

2. Combine milk, egg substitute, sugar, 2 teaspoons maple syrup, vanilla, and cinnamon in medium bowl. Stir in bread. Spoon evenly into prepared custard cups. Place cups in prepared pan.

3. Bake 40 minutes or until bread pudding is set. Drizzle remaining 1 teaspoon syrup over pudding. Serve immediately.

Makes 4 servings

COCOA

Naturally unsweetened and nearly fat free, cocoa powder adds wonderful chocolate taste, as well as health benefits, to low-calorie foods. Cocoa powder is made by removing most of the fat (cocoa butter) from the cocoa bean. This leaves rich, sugar-free chocolate flavor that's ready to use in all sorts of guilt-free homemade treats.

NUTRIENTS PER SERVING:

Cocoa powder, 1 tablespoon
Calories: 12
Protein: 1g
Total fat: 0.5g
Saturated fat: 0g
Cholesterol: 0mg
Carbohydrate: 3g
Dietary fiber: 2g
Sodium: 0mg
Potassium: 82mg
Calcium: 7mg
Iron: 0.8 mg
Magnesium: 27mg
Phosphorus: 40mg
Copper: 0.2mg

BENEFITS:

Cocoa powder is a concentrated source of plant nutrients called flavanols. Recent research indicates that flavanols can have beneficial effects on insulin sensitivity, as well as on blood pressure and the health of blood vessels, all of which help lower the risks of heart attack, stroke, and diabetes. Cocoa powder also provides fiber, iron, magnesium, phosphorus, potassium, and copper.

HOW TO SELECT AND STORE:

Natural cocoa powder is a light brown color and more acidic than Dutch process cocoa, which is a darker reddish brown color. Keep cocoa powder in an opaque, airtight container in a cool, dark place. It will last up to two years. Don't mistake cocoa powder for hot cocoa mix, which blends cocoa powder with powdered milk and sugar. Consuming large amounts of sweetened cocoa mix can have negative effects.

TIPS:

Cocoa powder is most often used in baked goods, such as brownies and cakes, or in low-fat puddings and beverages. When baking with cocoa powder, keep in mind that natural cocoa can create the rise in batter due to its high acid content, while Dutch process cocoa needs baking powder to create the same effect. Add unsweetened cocoa powder to water or low-fat milk to make a delicious diabetic drink.

INDIVIDUAL TIRAMISU CUPS

4 whole ladyfingers, broken into bite-size pieces

6 tablespoons cold strong coffee

2 packets sugar substitute

½ teaspoon vanilla

½ cup thawed frozen fat-free whipped topping

1½ teaspoons unsweetened cocoa powder

1 tablespoon sliced almonds

1. Place half the ladyfinger pieces in each of two 6-ounce custard cups. Set aside.

2. Combine coffee, sugar substitute, and vanilla in small bowl. Stir until sugar substitute is dissolved. Spoon 3 tablespoons of coffee mixture over each serving of ladyfinger pieces.

NUTRIENTS PER SERVING:

Tiramisu, ½ cup
Calories: 148
Calories from fat: 28%
Total fat: 5g
Saturated fat: 1g
Protein: 4g
Cholesterol: 80mg
Carbohydrate: 22g
Dietary fiber: 1g
Sodium: 43mg
Dietary exchanges:
1½ Starch, 1 Fat

3. Place whipped topping in small bowl. Fold in cocoa until blended. Spoon topping evenly over ladyfingers. Cover with plastic wrap and refrigerate for at least 2 hours.

4. Meanwhile, heat small skillet over medium high heat. Add almonds and toast 2 to 3 minutes or until golden, stirring constantly. Remove from heat; cool completely.

5. Sprinkle almonds over desserts just before serving.

Makes 2 servings

COFFEE

Best loved for the caffeine "buzz" it provides, emerging research suggests that coffee may offer a protection against type 2 diabetes, an even greater reason to down this popular beverage.

BENEFITS:

A promising, but so far unexplained, scientific observation is that coffee drinkers are less likely to develop diabetes. But even for those who already have the disease, coffee may offer benefits. Both regular and decaf coffee contain minerals such as chromium and magnesium that help the body use insulin. Both minerals are rich in antioxidants, which help protect the vulnerable heart and blood vessels. Plus, plain black coffee is a great choice for anyone who is diet-conscious.

HOW TO SELECT AND STORE:

You'll find myriad coffee selections at the store—from whole to ground, mild- to full-bodied, caffeinated or decaffeinated to instant and flavored. Choose the form and flavor depending on your preparation and your taste preferences. Store coffee beans or ground coffee in an airtight container in a cool, dry place. Whole beans should be used within a week or ground coffee within a few days. For long-term storage, keep coffee in the freezer.

NUTRIENTS PER SERVING:

Coffee, 1 cup brewed
Calories: 2
Protein: 0g
Total fat: 0g
Saturated fat: 0g
Cholesterol: 0mg
Carbohydrate: 0g
Dietary fiber: 0g
Sodium: 5mg
Potassium: 116mg
Magnesium: 7mg
Calcium: 5mg
Folate: 5mcg

TIPS:

Beware of coffee drinks loaded with sugary syrups, whole milk, and whipped cream, which can add loads of calories and fat. Coffee is a wonderful flavor enhancer and adds depth to various recipes, from desserts to main dishes, including chilis, pasta sauces and marinades, or glazes for meats.

CORIANDER

Coriander is both an herb and a spice since its leaves and seeds are used as a seasoning. Fresh coriander leaves are more commonly known as cilantro. The fruit of the coriander plant has seeds, which can be dried and used as a spice.

BENEFITS:

Both coriander and cilantro leaves are very low in calories and carbohydrates. Since they have less than 20 calories and have 5 grams or less of carbohydrate, both are considered "free foods" by the American Diabetes Association. Coriander seeds contain an array of phytonutrients—natural substances found in plants that help protect the plants from disease. In humans, phytonutrients have numerous health-promoting properties.

HOW TO SELECT AND STORE:

Ripe coriander seeds are a yellow-brown color. Keep coriander seeds and powder in an opaque, tightly sealed container in a cool, dark, dry place. Coriander powder keeps for about five months, while whole coriander seeds keep for about a year. The fresh leaves of the coriander plant (cilantro) should be a deep green color. Store fresh coriander/cilantro in the refrigerator. Whole coriander plants will remain fresh up to one week; the leaves (cilantro) will last up to three days.

NUTRIENTS PER SERVING:

Coriander seed, 1 teaspoon
Calories: 5
Protein: 0g
Total fat: 0g
Saturated fat: 0g
Cholesterol: 0mg
Carbohydrate: 1g
Dietary fiber: 1g
Sodium: 1mg
Magnesium: 6mg
Potassium: 23mg
Copper: 18mcg
Phosphorus: 7mg

TIPS:

Coriander seeds have a slight citrus flavor. You can use whole seeds or coriander powder in food. Cilantro is often featured in Latin American cuisine. Wash fresh cilantro right before using. Cilantro makes an excellent addition to salsas, soups, and sauces.

Avocado Salsa

1 medium avocado, peeled and diced

1 cup chopped seeded peeled cucumber

1 cup chopped onion

1 Anaheim chili, seeded and chopped*

½ cup chopped fresh tomato

2 tablespoons chopped fresh cilantro

½ teaspoon salt

¼ teaspoon hot pepper sauce

Chili peppers can sting and irritate skin. Wear rubber gloves when handling peppers and do not touch eyes. Wash hands after handling chili peppers.

NUTRIENTS PER SERVING:

Salsa, 2 tablespoons
Calories: 13
Calories from fat: 60%
Protein: <1g
Total fat: 1g
Saturated fat: <1g
Cholesterol: 0mg
Carbohydrate: 1g
Dietary fiber: <1g
Sodium: 38mg
Dietary exchanges: Free

1. Combine avocado, cucumber, onion, chili, tomato, cilantro, salt, and hot pepper sauce in medium bowl; mix well.

2. Refrigerate, covered, at least 1 hour to allow flavors to blend. Serve as dip or condiment.

Makes about 32 servings (4 cups)

COTTAGE CHEESE

Cottage cheese has gotten a bad rap as a standard diet food, but it has many uses besides a boring breakfast. It makes a great nutritious swap for the unhealthy ingredients found in many favorite dishes.

BENEFITS:

Cottage cheese is considered a dairy option in a traditional diabetic meal plan, but it's lower in carbohydrates and higher in protein than milk and yogurt. It provides long-lasting energy with little impact on blood sugar levels. Plus, it makes a great meat alternative, as the protein in cottage cheese is high quality. Select a fat-free or low-fat version, and this dieting staple can help you feel satisfied on fewer calories and less fat, which is good news for those who need to lose weight.

HOW TO SELECT AND STORE:

Choose low-fat (1%) or fat-free cottage cheese for fewer calories and fat than whole milk (4%) cottage cheese. It comes in small, medium, or large curd, which does not affect its nutrition profile. You can buy cottage cheese flavored, such as with chives or pineapple. Cottage cheese is perishable and must be stored in the refrigerator.

TIPS:

The flavor of cottage cheese goes well with fresh vegetables, such as tomatoes and bell peppers, and with fruits, such as pineapple and berries. Low-fat or fat-free cottage cheese makes a useful ingredient in various recipes. Use it to replace higher-fat cream cheese in desserts like cheesecakes and in dips. It also works great in place of high-fat cheeses in pasta dishes, such as lasagna or stuffed shells, and in egg-based dishes, such as quiches or frittatas.

NUTRIENTS PER SERVING:

Cottage cheese, ½ cup low-fat (1%)

Calories: 81
Protein: 14g
Total fat: 1g
Saturated fat: 0.5g
Cholesterol: 5mg
Carbohydrate: 3g
Dietary fiber: 0g
Sodium: 460mg
Potassium: 95mg
Calcium: 69mg
Vitamin A: 46 IU
Folate: 14mcg

CRANBERRIES

Cranberries make a colorful addition to holiday tables, but their tart taste and amazing health benefits can be enjoyed year round.

BENEFITS:

Cranberries contain phytonutrients that prevent certain bacteria from sticking to the walls of the urinary tract, thus helping to prevent or treat urinary tract infections. This same antibacterial effect may also help prevent gum disease and stomach ulcers, both commonly caused by bacteria. In addition, cranberries contain fiber as well as significant amounts of antioxidants and other phytonutrients that may help protect against heart disease, cancer, and eye diseases.

HOW TO SELECT AND STORE:

Fresh cranberries are at their peak from October to December. Choose bags of fresh cranberries that are firm, brightly colored, and unshriveled. They can be refrigerated, tightly wrapped, for at least two months, or frozen for up to a year. Select cranberry juice drinks with the least amount of added sugar. Because the pure juice is so tart, cranberry juice blends offer a 100% juice option without added sugar. Dried cranberries are also a good addition to your pantry.

NUTRIENTS PER SERVING:

Cranberries, ½ cup whole, raw
Calories: 23
Protein: 0g
Total fat: 0g
Saturated fat: 0g
Cholesterol: 0mg
Carbohydrate: 6g
Dietary fiber: 2g
Sodium: 1mg
Calcium: 4mg
Potassium: 43mg
Vitamin C: 7mg

TIPS:

This tart fruit can be baked into pies, cobblers, and quick breads or used in chutneys or salsas to complement poultry and pork dishes. Dried cranberries add sweetness and chewiness to salads, cereals, and cookies. Use cranberry juice blends in healthy smoothie recipes. Just be mindful of the sugar content when eating or drinking cranberry products.

CUCUMBER

Cucumber is light and refreshing, with its green skin, mild and crisp flesh, and tender seeds. Whether eaten alone or added to sandwiches or salads, this low-calorie, filling food is a great choice for any diet.

BENEFITS:

Because cucumbers are approximately 95 percent water, they are very low in calories. With such high water and low carbohydrate contents, cucumbers add low-calorie bulk and satisfying crunch to meals without having much effect on blood sugar levels.

HOW TO SELECT AND STORE:

Cucumbers are available year-round. Choose firm cucumbers with smooth, brightly colored skins. If you plan to eat the seeds, avoid larger cucumbers. As the fruit matures, the seeds grow larger and develop a bitter taste. Smaller cucumbers are used to make pickles. Store whole cucumbers, unwashed in a plastic bag, in the refrigerator for up to ten days. Cut cucumbers can be refrigerated, tightly wrapped, for up to five days.

NUTRIENTS PER SERVING:

Cucumber, ½ cup raw
Calories: 8
Protein: 0g
Total fat: 0g
Saturated fat: 0g
Cholesterol: 0mg
Carbohydrate: 2g
Dietary fiber: <1g
Sodium: 0mg
Potassium: 75mg
Calcium: 8mg
Iron: 0.2mg
Vitamin A: 55 IU
Vitamin C: 2mg
Folate: 4mcg

TIPS:

Wash cucumbers thoroughly just before using. Supermarket cucumbers are covered with an edible wax to protect from moisture loss. If you prefer not to eat the wax, peel the cucumber or use a produce rinse to remove the wax. Sliced cucumber makes a refreshing snack with a lower fat dip. Add them to salads for a delightful crunch. Try an Indian-inspired salad with cucumbers, fresh herbs, and plain yogurt. Cucumber makes an excellent main ingredient in a light, low-calorie cold soup. Be adventurous—pickle your own cucumbers.

DARK CHOCOLATE

Being diabetic doesn't mean giving up chocolate! Moderate amounts of dark chocolate can fit into your meal plan without sending blood sugar soaring.

BENEFITS:

Unlike other candies or sweet foods, dark chocolate has little effect on blood sugar. It contains antioxidants, essential minerals, and plant nutrients called flavanols that help protect the heart by lowering blood pressure and improving circulation. Protecting the heart is important for people with diabetes, since the disease increases the risk of cardiovascular disease. Still, moderation is essential, as dark chocolate is high in calories and saturated fat. To get the most benefit without overdoing calories, enjoy no more than 1 or 2 ounces per week.

NUTRIENTS PER SERVING:

Dark chocolate, 1 ounce
Calories: 154
Protein: 1g
Total fat: 9g
Saturated fat: 5g
Cholesterol: 2mg
Carbohydrate: 17g
Dietary fiber: 2g
Sodium: 6mg
Potassium: 160mg
Calcium: 16mg
Iron: 2.3mg
Magnesium: 43mg
Copper: 0.3mg
Phosphorus: 60mg

HOW TO SELECT AND STORE:

Dark chocolate is available in varying levels of "darkness," depending on the percentage of cocoa. For example, 60 percent cocoa content means that 40 percent of the product is made up of sugar, vanilla, and other ingredients. The higher the percentage of cocoa, the less sweet and more bitter it will taste. Dark chocolate includes semisweet and bittersweet varieties. Store dark chocolate, tightly wrapped, in a cool, dry place. Warmer temperatures will cause grayish streaks and blotches, which do not affect flavor.

TIPS:

Dark chocolate is best enjoyed on its own. It can be used in baking, in a variety of desserts, or simply as a garnish for a low-calorie dessert.

EGGPLANT

Filling and low in calories, this versatile vegetable is part of many popular ethnic dishes, including Indian curries, Greek moussaka, Middle Eastern baba ghanoush, and French ratatouille.

BENEFITS:

Eggplant is a decent source of fiber and potassium, but what makes it an especially appropriate addition to diabetes meal plans is that it's low in carbohydrates, so it doesn't cause spikes in blood sugar. It's also low in calories, so it can assist weight-loss efforts. Eggplant's meaty texture and flavor make it perfect for low-fat meatless dishes loaded with nutrient-rich grains, legumes, and vegetables.

HOW TO SELECT AND STORE:

Choose eggplants that are small, firm, and with thin skins. Larger ones tend to be seedy, tough, and bitter. The skin should range in color from deep purple to light violet or white. Eggplant is best used within a few days, but may be refrigerated for up to a week.

TIPS:

Eggplant can be eaten with or without the skin; use a potato peeler to remove the skin. To help reduce the bitterness, slice eggplant, sprinkle with salt, and let it stand for 30 minutes. Then, drain it and blot dry before cooking. Eggplant can be baked, roasted, grilled, steamed, or sautéed. Eggplant is done when it can be pierced easily with a fork. It tends to absorb fats easily, so go easy on fatty ingredients. Eggplant makes a tasty addition to stir-fry, lasagna, and pasta dishes. Or it can be stuffed with other flavorful veggies and baked.

NUTRIENTS PER SERVING:

Eggplant, ½ cup cooked
Calories: 17
Protein: 0g
Total fat: 0g
Saturated fat: 0g
Cholesterol: 0g
Carbohydrate: 4g
Dietary fiber: 1g
Sodium: 0mg
Potassium: 60mg
Calcium: 3mg
Iron: 0.1mg
Vitamin A: 18 IU
Vitamin C: 1mg
Folate: 7mcg

EGGS

For years, eggs have been cast in a negative light. But the incredible egg is quite beneficial. Eating eggs is a great way to start your day, as they are rich in protein and many nutrients.

BENEFITS:

Even though eggs are high in cholesterol, research indicates they can be a healthy addition to a diabetes meal plan. Eggs offer 13 essential vitamins and minerals, high-quality protein, healthy unsaturated fats, and protective antioxidants, all for about 75 calories per egg. Enjoying eggs at breakfast has been shown to help control both hunger and blood sugar levels. But what about all that cholesterol? It turns out the saturated fat in the foods we eat, far more than the cholesterol content, is what jacks up cholesterol levels. And eggs are actually rather low in saturated fats. Keep in mind that pairing eggs with bacon and sausage—foods loaded with saturated fat—will not favor your cholesterol levels.

HOW TO SELECT AND STORE:

Choose eggs that are clean and not cracked, and always check the "sell by" date for freshness. Brown eggs and those labeled as "farm-laid" or "free-range" are no more nutritious. However, eggs from hens fed a diet rich in omega-3 fatty acids will contain more of this healthy fat. Store eggs in the carton in the refrigerator for up to three weeks.

TIPS:

Eggs are a versatile food on their own. They also serve as an essential ingredient in recipes—helping baked goods to rise, binding ingredients in casseroles, thickening custards and sauces, and emulsifying mayonnaise and salad dressings, to name a few.

FENNEL

This vegetable may be a stranger to many, but it shouldn't be! Fennel provides wonderful flavor and texture to many dishes, as well as plenty of nutrients.

BENEFITS:

Fennel provides several essential nutrients without contributing much in the way of carbohydrates or calories, making it a good food to include in your diet if you have type 2 diabetes. In addition to offering vitamin C, calcium, iron, and folate, fennel is a good source of fiber and potassium, which is great for the many people with diabetes who also have heart disease. The potassium helps lower high blood pressure and the fiber helps lower blood cholesterol. The fiber also prevents wild spikes in blood sugar levels.

HOW TO SELECT AND STORE:

Select fennel that has a whitish bulb, white to pale green stalks, and light green and delicate leaves. The bulb should be firm and without signs of browning or drying. Store fresh fennel in a plastic bag in the crisper drawer for up to five days. Fennel seeds are available both ground and whole in the spice section of the supermarket.

NUTRIENTS PER SERVING:

Fennel, ½ cup raw
Calories: 13
Protein: 1g
Total fat: 0g
Saturated fat: 0g
Cholesterol: 0mg
Carbohydrate: 3g
Dietary fiber: 1g
Sodium: 25mg
Potassium: 180mg
Calcium: 21mg
Iron: 0.3mg
Vitamin A: 58 IU
Vitamin C: 5mg
Folate: 12mcg

TIPS:

All parts of fennel can be used—stalks, leaves, and bulb. Rinse fennel well to remove dirt from the bulb and between the stalks. Fennel can be enjoyed raw in salads, braised or sautéed as a side dish, or in soups and stews. The fragrant greens can be used as a garnish and flavor enhancer. Fennel seeds are often added to meatballs or meat loaves for an Italian flavor.

FLAX SEED

Many people had never heard of flax seed until recent years. Its popularity has increased immensely because of its powerful health benefits. To unlock its potential, flax seed must be ground before eating.

BENEFITS:

Flax seed's nutrient profile makes it ideal for people with diabetes. It's high in fiber, which helps steady blood sugar levels, but very low in the other types of carbohydrates— the sugars and starches that cause blood sugar to shoot up. It also carries a substantial dose of omega-3 fatty acids, an essential polyunsaturated fat the body can't make for itself. Recent research suggests omega-3 fats may improve insulin sensitivity and help prevent diabetic retinopathy.

HOW TO SELECT AND STORE:

Flax seed is available whole or ground into meal. Because ground flax will go rancid quickly, it's better to buy whole flax seed and grind it yourself, which takes seconds in a food processor or blender. Once ground, flax seed should be stored in an airtight container in the freezer and used within a few weeks. Whole flax seed stays fresh for up to a year if stored in a cool, dark, dry place.

NUTRIENTS PER SERVING:
Flax seed, 1 tablespoon ground
Calories: 37
Protein: 1g
Total fat: 3g
Saturated fat: 0g
Cholesterol: 0mg
Carbohydrate: 2g
Dietary fiber: 2g
Sodium: 0mg
Potassium: 60mg
Calcium: 18mg
Iron: 0.4mg
Phosphorus: 45mg
Magnesium: 27mg

TIPS:

Flax seed has a pleasant nutty flavor, but it's almost undetectable when added to many foods. A few tablespoons of ground flax seed can be added to breads, muffins, cookies, and pancakes. Sprinkle over cottage cheese, yogurt, cereal, or salads. Add it to smoothies for a boost. It can also be cooked into meat loaf, meatballs, and casseroles.

GARBANZO BEANS

Also known as chickpeas, garbanzo beans have a nutty taste and a buttery texture. This versatile legume is the main ingredient in many Middle Eastern and Indian dishes and is the perfect addition to a diabetic meal plan.

BENEFITS:

Garbanzo beans are chock-full of fiber, which helps keep you feeling full longer. While containing conventional nutrients like vitamin C, vitamin E, and beta-carotene, garbanzo beans also contain concentrated supplies of antioxidant phytonutrients, which have health-promoting properties. Recent research indicates that garbanzo beans may help regulate blood sugar, lower harmful LDL cholesterol levels, and reduce the risk of heart disease.

HOW TO SELECT AND STORE:

Garbanzo beans are available dried or canned. Store dried garbanzo beans in an airtight container in a cool, dark, dry place for up to a year. Cooked garbanzo beans will keep fresh in the refrigerator for three days.

TIPS:

Garbanzo beans are commonly found in hummus, falafel, and curry. But they can also be used in vegetable soup, in a pasta dish, with brown rice, or sprinkled over a salad. Rinse canned garbanzo beans before using to reduce sodium. After rinsing dried beans, you can presoak them before cooking to reduce cooking time. Cook beans on the stovetop or in a pressure cooker, or according to recipe instructions.

> ## NUTRIENTS PER SERVING:
>
> *Garbanzo beans (chickpeas), ½ cup cooked*
> **Calories:** 148
> **Protein:** 8g
> **Total fat:** 2g
> **Saturated fat:** 0g
> **Cholesterol:** 0mg
> **Carbohydrate:** 25g
> **Dietary fiber:** 7g
> **Sodium:** 6mg
> **Calcium:** 39mg
> **Potassium:** 248mg
> **Magnesium:** 35mg
> **Phosphorus:** 126mg
> **Vitamin B$_6$:** 0.1mg
> **Vitamin K:** 4mcg
> **Zinc:** 1mg

HUMMUS with PITA CHIPS

1 can (about 15 ounces) garbanzo beans (chickpeas), rinsed and drained

3 tablespoons lemon juice

4½ teaspoons tahini*

½ teaspoon ground cumin

¼ teaspoon salt

¼ teaspoon black pepper

½ cup chopped seeded tomato

⅓ cup chopped red onion

⅓ cup chopped celery

⅓ cup chopped seeded cucumber

⅓ cup chopped green or red bell pepper

2 pita bread rounds

Tahini, a paste made from sesame seeds, is available in ethnic sections of supermarkets, Middle Eastern markets, and health food stores.

NUTRIENTS PER SERVING:

3 tablespoons hummus and 4 pita chips

Calories: 235
Calories from fat: 15%
Protein: 11g
Total fat: 4g
Saturated fat: <1g
Cholesterol: 0mg
Carbohydrate: 41g
Dietary fiber: 8g
Sodium: 252mg
Dietary exchanges:
½ Vegetable, 2 Starch, ½ Fat

1. Combine garbanzo beans (chickpeas), lemon juice, tahini, cumin, salt, and black pepper in food processor or blender; process until smooth. If mixture is too thick to spread, add water, 1 tablespoon at a time, until desired consistency is reached.

2. Spoon hummus into serving bowl. Top with tomato, onion, celery, cucumber, and bell pepper.

3. Preheat broiler. Split pitas horizontally in half to form 4 rounds. Cut each round into 6 wedges. Place on baking sheet; broil 3 minutes or until crisp.

4. Serve hummus with pita wedges.

Makes 6 servings

GARLIC

If you don't already love garlic's pungent flavor, you should. Not only does it add a ton of flavor when used in cooking, it has wonderful health benefits, too.

BENEFITS:

Whenever garlic is crushed or cooked, a substance called allicin is formed, providing garlic's distinctive aroma and flavor. Allicin may also play a significant role in heart health, which is important for people with diabetes, who are at a higher risk for heart disease. Studies indicate garlic may help lower high blood pressure and slow the hardening of arteries, which often leads to heart disease or stroke. Garlic also thins the blood, which may help prevent blood clots, but also could cause problems during trauma or surgery. Your best bet is to consult your doctor on this.

HOW TO SELECT AND STORE:

Pink-skinned garlic is sweeter and keeps longer than white garlic. Large elephant garlic is milder in flavor and can be used similarly to leeks. Choose loose garlic that is firm to the touch with no visible damp or brown spots. Jarred garlic and garlic powder are convenient, but not as flavorful as fresh. If using garlic salt, keep in mind that it contains a lot of sodium. Store garlic in a cool, dark, dry spot. It will last anywhere from a few weeks to a few months.

TIPS:

Use pressed garlic when you want full-force garlic flavor to come through, and minced garlic when you want milder flavor. For a buttery flavor, bake whole cloves until tender. The longer garlic is cooked, the milder the flavor.

GRAPEFRUIT

Grapefruit's juiciness, tart flavor, and filling fiber make it a wonderful food to include in your meal plan. It's low in calories, too!

BENEFITS:

Grapefruit's soluble fiber helps stabilize blood sugar and lower cholesterol, which is often elevated in people with diabetes. It's rich in vitamin A, a vitamin essential for fending off infections and preventing vision problems, two categories of disease that are more common when blood sugar levels are consistently high. Grapefruit is also a good source of vitamin C and beta-carotene, which research has shown can help prevent cataracts and macular degeneration. Because grapefruit and its juice may interfere with the actions of certain medications, be sure to read labels carefully and consult your physician and pharmacist.

NUTRIENTS PER SERVING:

Grapefruit, ½ medium
Calories: 41
Protein: 1g
Total fat: 0g
Saturated fat: 0g
Cholesterol: 0mg
Carbohydrate: 10g
Dietary fiber: 1.5g
Sodium: 0mg
Potassium: 180mg
Calcium: 15mg
Iron: 0.1mg
Vitamin A: 1,187 IU
Vitamin C: 44mg
Folate: 13mcg

HOW TO SELECT AND STORE:

Choose grapefruit that feels heavy, and avoid those that are soft or mushy, or oblong rather than round. The difference in taste among white, red, and pink varieties of grapefruit is minimal; they are equally sweet (and tart). Store grapefruit in your refrigerator's crisper drawer; they'll keep for up to two months.

TIPS:

Wash grapefruit before cutting to prevent bacteria on the skin from being introduced to the inside. You might want to bring grapefruit to room temperature before you juice or slice it for better flavor. Beyond the typical halved grapefruit at breakfast, try peeling and eating it out of hand for a juicy, mouthwatering snack.

GRAPES

Grapes are a fast, portable, and diabetic-friendly snack. They offer the same hand-to-mouth action that other sweet snacks provide, but with fewer calories.

BENEFITS:

Grapes are a refreshing low-calorie substitute for high-fat, calorie-filled snacks and desserts and are perfect for when you're craving something sweet. High in water and a respectable source of fiber, grapes are filling and provide only about 60 calories per bunch of 15 to 17 grapes. Grapes also contain a collection of powerful phytonutrients that may help fight heart disease.

HOW TO SELECT AND STORE:

When buying grapes, look for clusters with plump, well-colored fruit attached to pliable, green stems. Avoid soft, wrinkled grapes or those with browned areas around the stem. Good color is the key to flavor. The sweetest green grapes are yellow-green in color, red varieties that are predominantly crimson-red will have the best flavor, and blue-purple varieties taste best if their color is deep and rich, almost black. Most are available seedless. Stored unwashed in the fridge up to a week.

NUTRIENTS PER SERVING:

Grapes, ½ cup
Calories: 31
Protein: 0g
Total fat: 0g
Saturated fat: 0g
Cholesterol: 0mg
Carbohydrate: 8g
Dietary fiber: <1g
Sodium: 0mg
Potassium: 90mg
Calcium: 6mg
Iron: 0.1mg
Vitamin A: 46 IU
Vitamin C: 2mg
Folate: 2mcg

TIPS:

Rinse grape clusters just before eating. Chilling enhances their flavor. Frozen grapes make a popular summer treat. Cold sliced grapes taste great in low-fat yogurt. Skewer grapes, banana slices, apple chunks, and pineapple cubes and serve with a low-fat creamy dip. Or brush skewers with a combination of honey, lemon, and ground nutmeg.

GREEK YOGURT

This Mediterranean-style yogurt is not only creamier and thicker than regular yogurt, but contains almost double the protein with fewer carbohydrates, making it a winner for people with diabetes.

BENEFITS:

If you're looking for a healthy, calcium-rich dairy food but need to watch your carbohydrate intake, Greek yogurt is a great choice. While regular yogurts have 15–17 grams of carbohydrates per 4-ounce serving, Greek yogurt averages around 9 grams, and some brands have even less. Because it is rich in lean protein, Greek yogurt provides long-lasting energy without a surge in blood sugar levels. A triple-straining process that removes more whey (liquid) is what makes Greek yogurt so creamy. It also lowers the lactose content, making this yogurt easier for some people to digest. Greek yogurt contains about 50 percent less sodium than regular yogurt, making it a better choice if you're also battling high blood pressure. Like regular varieties, Greek yogurt provides healthy bacteria, or probiotics, to help keep your immune system humming.

NUTRIENTS PER SERVING:

Greek yogurt, ½ cup nonfat
Calories: 80
Protein: 11g
Total fat: 0g
Saturated fat: 0g
Cholesterol: 0mg
Carbohydrate: 9g
Dietary fiber: 0g
Sodium: 45mg
Potassium: 160mg
Calcium: 150mg

HOW TO SELECT AND STORE:

Greek yogurt is a newcomer to the yogurt aisle, but its growing popularity is bringing it to most supermarkets. Like regular yogurt, it is available in nonfat, low-fat, and whole milk varieties. Flavors include plain, vanilla, fruit varieties, and Mediterranean-influenced honey. Store Greek yogurt in the refrigerator and use within two weeks.

TIPS:

Greek yogurt can be enjoyed straight from the carton or used as a base in salad dressings, dips, sauces, smoothies, ice creams, and desserts.

GREEN BEANS

Green beans, also known as snap beans, are a great vegetable choice for people with diabetes. Not only are they low in carbohydrates, their crunchy texture makes them a pleasure to eat—a double bonus.

BENEFITS:

Green beans are low in calories and carbohydrates, so they're less likely to have a negative effect on your blood sugar or waistline. They provide essential vitamins, minerals, and fiber. Green beans contain chromium, a mineral that is known to enhance the action of insulin. Green beans are also rich in carotenoids beta-carotene and lutein. Lutein may help protect eyes from the vision complications associated with diabetes.

HOW TO SELECT AND STORE:

Fresh green beans are at their peak from May to October, but frozen green beans come very close nutritionally. Canned green beans may lose some vitamins during processing, and typically contain more sodium. Choose fresh green beans that are slender, crisp, brightly colored, and without blemishes. Store them in a plastic bag in the refrigerator for up to five days.

NUTRIENTS PER SERVING:

Green beans, ½ cup cooked
Calories: 22
Protein: 1g
Total fat: 0g
Saturated fat: 0g
Cholesterol: 0mg
Carbohydrate: 5g
Dietary fiber: 2g
Sodium: 0mg
Potassium: 90mg
Calcium: 28mg
Chromium: 1mcg
Iron: 0.4mg
Vitamin A: 438 IU
Vitamin C: 6mg
Folate: 21mcg

TIPS:

Fresh or frozen green beans can be steamed lightly on the stove or in the microwave just until tender-crisp. Rinse canned green beans to lower the sodium and heat gently to prevent them from getting mushy. Lightly season with herbs, or sprinkle with toasted nuts. Add green beans to soups or casseroles or enjoy raw with a low-fat dip.

JICAMA

Don't be a stranger to this root vegetable. Often referred to as a Mexican potato, jicama is refreshingly crisp and crunchy, with a sweet, nutty flavor, and radish-like texture.

BENEFITS:

Foods like jicama that have a high water content and ample fiber help prevent sudden, large shifts in blood sugar levels. Such foods also fill you up without piling on calories and fats, helping with weight-loss. Plus, jicama provides vitamin C, which research suggests can help protect arteries from damage that can lead to heart attacks and strokes.

HOW TO SELECT AND STORE:

Jicama is available in most supermarkets from November through May. Select jicama that is firm and unblemished with a slightly silky sheen. It should not feel soft or have bruises or wrinkles, which signal that it's been stored too long. Jicama can be stored for up to two weeks in a plastic bag in the refrigerator.

TIPS:

Jicama is a versatile vegetable that adds a crisp texture and nutty sweetness to foods. It also tends to take on flavors of foods that it accompanies. The thin skin of jicama should be peeled before eating or cooking. Cut the flesh of jicama into cubes or sticks and add it to salads, salsa, or coleslaw. It can also be added to stir-fries or roasted with other vegetables. Simply enjoy it alone or with a low-fat dip. For a refreshing salad, combine cubed jicama, sliced cucumber, and orange sections, and sprinkle with chili powder, salt, and a drizzle of fresh lemon juice.

NUTRIENTS PER SERVING:

Jicama, ½ cup raw
Calories: 25
Protein: <1g
Total fat: 0g
Saturated fat: 0g
Cholesterol: 0mg
Carbohydrate: 6g
Dietary fiber: 3g
Sodium: 5mg
Potassium: 100mg
Calcium: 8mg
Iron: 0.4mg
Vitamin A: 14 IU
Vitamin C: 13mg
Folate: 8mcg

KIWI

The brown, fuzzy outside of kiwi hides a gorgeous emerald green interior loaded with nutrition. The sweet-tart taste and distinctive color of kiwi can jazz up salads, desserts, and even drinks.

BENEFITS:

Just one medium kiwi provides an entire day's worth of vitamin C, which may protect arteries, including those feeding the heart and brain, from damage. Kiwi also packs potassium for healthy blood pressure and the antioxidants lutein and zeaxanthin, which safeguard the eyes. The fruit's flesh contains soluble fiber, which helps reduce blood cholesterol, and its little black seeds contribute insoluble fiber.

HOW TO SELECT AND STORE:

Kiwis are available year-round. Choose those that are fragrant and fairly firm but give under gentle pressure. Firm kiwis need about a week to ripen at room temperature. Speed ripening by placing them in a closed paper bag for one to two days. Ripe kiwis keep for one to two weeks in the refrigerator.

NUTRIENTS PER SERVING:

Kiwi, 1 medium
Calories: 42
Protein: 1g
Total fat: 0g
Saturated fat: 0g
Cholesterol: 0mg
Carbohydrate: 10g
Dietary fiber: 2g
Sodium: 0mg
Calcium: 23mg
Potassium: 215mg
Iron: 0.2mg
Vitamin A: 60 IU
Vitamin C: 64mg
Folate: 17mcg

TIPS:

With their brilliant green color and inner circle of tiny black seeds, sliced kiwis shine in fruit and vegetable salads. They don't even discolor when exposed to air. Most people prefer eating peeled kiwi, though the skin is edible. Just wash them and rub off the brown fuzz. For a handheld treat, cut an unpeeled kiwi in half and scoop out the flesh with a spoon. Since kiwi contains an enzyme that prevents gelatin from setting, you'll want to leave it out of molded salads.

LEMONS

Lemons' tart juice and zesty rind add life to everything from fish and vegetables to tea and water, helping to perk up the fresh, healthy foods in your diabetes meal plan.

NUTRIENTS PER SERVING:

Lemon, 1 medium
Calories: 24
Protein: <1g
Total fat: 0g
Saturated fat: 0g
Cholesterol: 0mg
Carbohydrate: 8g
Dietary fiber: 2.5g
Sodium: 0mg
Potassium: 115mg
Calcium: 22mg
Iron: 0.5mg
Vitamin A: 18 IU
Vitamin C: 45mg
Folate: 9mcg

BENEFITS:

Lemons are loaded with vitamin C, which is essential for controlling infections. That is especially important for people with diabetes, who are at increased risk for a variety of infections. As an antioxidant, vitamin C also helps fight inflammation, which is suspected of playing a role not only in the development of diabetes, but in its progression and complications. Lemons' zest, or outer skin, is rich in another antioxidant, rutin, which may help strengthen blood vessel walls and protect them from damage.

HOW TO SELECT AND STORE:

Look for firm, unblemished lemons that are heavy for their size—an indicator of juiciness. Thin-skinned fruits yield the most juice. Refrigerated, they keep for a month or two. Lemon varieties vary mostly in their skin thickness, juiciness, and number of seeds.

TIPS:

To get more juice from a lemon, bring it to room temperature, then roll back and forth under the palm of your hand before you cut and squeeze it. Another flavorful part of the fruit is its zest. Scrape off with a grater, knife, or zester, and use to enhance desserts and fruit salads. Wash lemons thoroughly before grating the peel or cutting into the flesh. Lemon adds a flavorful zing to fish and bean dishes, helping reduce the need for unhealthy sauces and seasonings.

LIMES

Using lime juice in cooking is an easy, healthy way to perk up any dish. Just add a splash with a few herbs, and your meal will be full of flavor, not calories.

BENEFITS:

Lime juice provides a ton of flavor for very few calories and carbohydrates. Limes also contain hefty amounts of vitamin C, helping the body fight infections. This is important for people with diabetes, as infections tend to develop more easily due to damage to the nerves and blood vessels by high blood sugar levels. Additionally, the powerful phytochemicals found in limes may help protect cells from damage that can lead to heart disease.

HOW TO SELECT AND STORE:

The Persian lime is the most common variety. The key lime, the main star in the tropical dessert, is small and round, while the Persian looks more like a green lemon. Key limes are generally more flavorful due to their acidity. Limes typically turn yellowish as they ripen. The greenest limes have the best flavor. Refrigerated, they keep for a month or two.

TIPS:

Lime juice can be used as a salt substitute for meat and fish dishes, and a splash of lime juice over fruit prevents discoloration while adding a zing of flavor. To get more juice from a lime, bring it to room temperature, then roll it back and forth under the palm of your hand before you cut and squeeze it. Lime peel is often used to add flavor to salads, dressings, and desserts.

NUTRIENTS PER SERVING:

Lime, 1 medium raw
Calories: 20
Protein: <1g
Total fat: 0g
Saturated fat: 0g
Cholesterol: 0mg
Carbohydrate: 7g
Dietary fiber: 2g
Sodium: 0mg
Potassium: 70mg
Calcium: 22mg
Iron: 0.4mg
Vitamin A: 34 IU
Vitamin C: 20mg
Folate: 5mcg

Yogurt Lime Tartlets

1 refrigerated pie crust (half of 14-ounce package)

1 cup plain nonfat Greek yogurt

2 tablespoons honey

1 egg, lightly beaten

Grated peel and juice of 1 lime

Additional grated lime peel (optional)

1. Preheat oven to 350°F. Spray 14 standard (2½-inch) muffin cups with nonstick cooking spray.

2. Unroll pie crust on work surface. Cut out circles with 3-inch round cookie cutter. Reroll scraps to cut out total of 14 circles. Press circles onto bottoms and up sides of prepared muffin cups.

NUTRIENTS PER SERVING:

1 tartlet
Calories: 97
Protein: 2g
Total fat: 5g
Saturated fat: 2g
Cholesterol: 13mg
Carbohydrate: 12g
Dietary fiber: 1g
Sodium: 78mg
Dietary exchanges:
1 Starch, 1 Fat

3. Stir yogurt, honey, egg, and grated peel and juice of 1 lime in medium bowl until well blended. Spoon 1 tablespoon mixture into each prepared muffin cup.

4. Bake 18 minutes or until set and crust is golden brown. Cool in pan on wire rack 5 minutes. Remove to wire rack; cool completely. Refrigerate at least 2 hours before serving. Garnish with additional grated lime peel.

Makes 14 tartlets

MANGO

No wonder the mango is sometimes called the king of fruits. It is beautiful, fragrant, and offers a wealth of nutrients along with a unique taste of tropical sweetness.

BENEFITS:

Mangoes are a superior source of beta-carotene, a vitamin-A precursor and antioxidant that helps maintain eye health—which is of special concern to people with diabetes. And just one mango provides almost an entire day's worth of vitamin C, itself a powerful antioxidant. Mangoes also contribute calcium, potassium, and magnesium; regularly consuming foods rich in these three minerals is associated with lower blood pressure.

HOW TO SELECT AND STORE:

There are more than 200 varieties of mangoes with colors ranging from yellow to bright red and orange. Choose those that feel firm, but yield to slight pressure. The color should have begun to change from green to yellow, orange, or red. You can speed the process by placing a mango in a paper bag for a few days. Mango is also available canned or frozen.

NUTRIENTS PER SERVING:

Mango, ½ medium raw
Calories: 101
Protein: 1g
Total fat: 0.5g
Saturated fat: 0g
Cholesterol: 0mg
Carbohydrate: 25g
Dietary fiber: 2.5g
Sodium: 0mg
Calcium: 18mg
Potassium: 280mg
Magnesium: 17mg
Vitamin A: 1,818 IU
Vitamin C: 61mg
Folate: 72mcg

TIPS:

The tricky part of preparing a mango is cutting the flesh away from the long flat pit in the center. The thicker part of mango flesh is on the flatter sides of the mango. Stand the mango on end and slice the fruit from stem to tip, coming as close as you can to the pit. Lay each mango cheek skin side down and score the flesh in a crosshatch pattern without cutting through the skin. Then turn the piece inside out. The cubes of mango will be easy to slice away.

MILK

Known best for its role in bone health and its high calcium and protein contents, milk's rich nutrients make it great for a diabetic diet.

BENEFITS:

Vitamin D has recently been found to not only play a role in bone health, but also in regulating blood sugar levels. A growing body of evidence indicates that a deficiency in vitamin D can increase the risk of type 2 diabetes as well as diabetes-related complications. Furthermore, people with diabetes who don't get enough vitamin D have close to double the risk of heart disease and a greater risk of heart attack and stroke than people with diabetes with adequate levels. Fortunately, it is easy to get vitamin D from fortified milk.

NUTRIENTS PER SERVING:

Milk, 1 cup fat-free, fortified with A and D
Calories: 83
Protein: 8g
Total fat: 0g
Saturated fat: 0g
Cholesterol: 5mg
Carbohydrate: 12g
Dietary fiber: 0g
Sodium: 105mg
Potassium: 380mg
Calcium: 299mg
Vitamin A: 500 IU
Vitamin D: 115 IU
Folate: 12mcg

HOW TO SELECT AND STORE:

Milk varies in the percentage of fat, from whole (4%) to reduced-fat (2%), low-fat (1%) and fat-free (skim). There are significant fat and calorie savings between whole and fat-free milk, but no difference in nutrient content. To capture the most benefit, choose milk fortified with vitamins A and D. All milk containers should have a "sell by" date and will stay fresh about seven days after this date. Avoid raw, unpasteurized milk, as it may carry harmful bacteria.

TIPS:

Milk tastes best when served icy cold. It is rich in protein, making it filling and satisfying—no matter how you enjoy it. Drink it alone as a snack or in a smoothie with your favorite fruits for a sweet, satisfying meal. Most recipes that call for milk, like soups and casseroles, work fine with lower fat milk varieties.

MUSHROOMS

Mushrooms can be enjoyed in countless ways, but their hearty texture makes them best enjoyed as a low-calorie meat substitute.

BENEFITS:

Mushrooms are essentially a "free food" in a diabetic diet, as they are very low in calories and carbohydrates. They are also virtually sodium-free and provide hefty amounts of potassium, which benefits people who also have high blood pressure. What makes mushrooms stand out is that they are the only source of vitamin D found in the produce aisle. Many varieties are also rich in selenium, an antioxidant mineral.

HOW TO SELECT AND STORE:

All supermarkets stock the white button mushroom, and many have expanded their selection to include other varieties such as shiitake, chanterelle, enoki, morel, oyster, Portobello, and the often dried Chinese wood-ear. Mushrooms like cool, humid, circulating air and need to be stored in a paper bag or ventilated container in your refrigerator, but not in the crisper drawer. Mushrooms last only a couple of days, but can still be used to impart flavor in cooking after they've turned brown.

NUTRIENTS PER SERVING:

Mushrooms, ½ cup cooked
Calories: 22
Protein: 2g
Total fat: 1g
Saturated fat: 0g
Cholesterol: 0mg
Carbohydrate: 4g
Dietary fiber: 2g
Sodium: 0mg
Potassium: 278mg
Calcium: 5mg
Iron: 1.4mg
Selenium: 9mcg
Niacin: 3.5mg
Riboflavin: 0.2mg

TIPS:

To clean, use a mushroom brush or wipe mushrooms with a damp cloth. Don't cut mushrooms until you're ready to use them. Mushrooms cook quickly. They'll absorb oil in cooking, so it's best to sauté mushrooms in broth or wine. Portobello mushrooms are good for grilling and can take the place of meat in many dishes, including burgers and meat loaves.

MUSTARD GREENS

Mustard greens and their cousins, beet, collard, dandelion, and turnip greens, are gaining recognition as nutrition powerhouses, having more antioxidants than many common fruits and vegetables. Peppery mustard greens are one of the most nutritious of all the leafy greens.

BENEFITS:

All leafy greens are loaded with powerful phytonutrients, and research shows an extra daily serving could help decrease the risk of type 2 diabetes and diabetes complications. Mustard greens are full of folate, beta-carotene, and vitamin C, all of which support the heart and blood vessels. They also contain soluble fiber, which helps lower blood cholesterol levels and fight hunger.

NUTRIENTS PER SERVING:

Mustard greens, ½ cup cooked
Calories: 10
Protein: 2g
Total fat: 0g
Saturated fat: 0g
Cholesterol: 0mg
Carbohydrate: 2g
Dietary fiber: 1.5g
Sodium: 10mg
Potassium: 140mg
Calcium: 52mg
Iron: 0.5mg
Vitamin A: 4,426 IU
Vitamin C: 18mg
Folate: 51mcg

HOW TO SELECT AND STORE:

Look for fresh mustard greens with crisp, dark green leaves. Choose small leaves and avoid those that are sunken, spotted, or discolored. Unwashed greens store best when wrapped in a damp paper towel in an airtight plastic bag in the refrigerator. They will last three to five days but should be eaten soon after purchase as they develop a strong bitter flavor over time. Mustard greens are also available frozen or canned and can be used in place of fresh in many dishes.

TIPS:

Wash greens well and remove tough stems. Mustard greens can be steamed, sautéed, or simmered until wilted. For a tasty side dish, simmer in broth and season with onion and garlic. Try mustard greens in stir-fries. Frozen or canned mustard greens work great in soups and stews.

MUSTARD SEEDS

Mustard isn't as sinful as it seems. Because mustard seeds are relatively low in carbohydrate and calories, they can be enjoyed without guilt.

BENEFITS:

Mustard seeds, which come from the mustard plant, have surprising health benefits. Mustard seeds contain phytonutrients. They are an excellent source of magnesium, a nutrient that helps lower high blood pressure. Mustard seeds also supply omega-3 fatty acids, manganese, phosphorus, copper, and thiamin (vitamin B_1).

HOW TO SELECT AND STORE:

Mustard seeds are sold either whole or as a ground powder. Whole seeds are available in white (which are actually yellow), brown, and black varieties. The darker the seed, the more pungent the taste. American yellow mustard is made with white seeds, while Dijon mustard is made with brown seeds. Both mustard powder and mustard seeds should be kept in a tightly sealed container in a cool, dark, dry place. Prepared mustard should be refrigerated.

TIPS:

You can use whole mustard seeds or mustard powder in cooking. To make your own mustard condiment, soak the seeds in water until softened. Grind the seeds into a paste using a mortar and pestle or blender, adding herbs and spices such as garlic, tarragon, turmeric, paprika, or pepper to taste. Try marinating chicken or salmon fillets with mustard. Add honey or cinnamon to mustard to create a sweet dipping sauce. Mix prepared mustard with a vinaigrette dressing and use on salads.

NUTRIENTS PER SERVING:

Mustard seeds, 1 teaspoon ground
Calories: 10
Protein: 1g
Total fat: 1g
Saturated fat: 0g
Cholesterol: 0mg
Carbohydrate: 1g
Dietary fiber: 0g
Sodium: 0mg
Calcium: 5mg
Potassium: 15mg
Magnesium: 7mg
Phosphorus: 17mg
Selenium: 4mcg

NECTARINES

For a delicious way to satisfy your sweet tooth, try a juicy nectarine. Named for its delicious nectar, this fruit is a wonderful low-calorie treat for people with diabetes.

BENEFITS:

The flesh of the nectarine is a rich source of soluble fiber, the kind that slows the absorption of sugar, preventing blood sugar levels from fluctuating. Nectarines' generous fiber content can also help lower blood cholesterol levels and may assist in blood pressure control. Additionally, nectarines can help prevent diabetes-related complications. They contain beta-carotene, an antioxidant that converts to vitamin A in the body, which plays an essential role in eye health.

NUTRIENTS PER SERVING:

Nectarine, 1 medium raw
Calories: 62
Protein: 2g
Total fat: 0g
Saturated fat: 0g
Cholesterol: 0mg
Carbohydrate: 15g
Dietary fiber: 2.5g
Sodium: 0mg
Potassium: 285mg
Calcium: 9mg
Vitamin A: 471 IU
Vitamin C: 8mg
Folate: 7mcg

HOW TO SELECT AND STORE:

Nectarines look like peaches without the fuzz, but you'll also find a white nectarine variation with lighter skin and flesh. Nectarines are at their best from mid-spring to early fall. Choose nectarines that are firm, yet give slightly to the touch. Avoid those with bruises or blemishes, as well as those that are hard or overly green. Slightly under-ripe nectarines will ripen at room temperature within a couple of days. Refrigerate to help slow ripening, but use within five days.

TIPS:

A ripe nectarine is a juicy treat, whether eaten out of hand or sliced from the pit. They make a delicious addition to salads and can be used in a variety of fresh or cooked desserts. The flesh will darken when exposed to air, so be sure to sprinkle with lemon juice to prevent browning when served in fresh salads or desserts.

OATMEAL

Oatmeal, the classic breakfast staple, is full of whole grain goodness. All oats—instant, quick, old-fashioned, or steel-cut—are beneficial for people with diabetes.

BENEFITS:

Oatmeal is known for its soluble fiber, which slows digestion and keeps blood sugar levels even. Choosing high-fiber foods like oatmeal can help decrease the risk of heart disease. One way it defends the heart is by lowering levels of total and LDL ("bad") cholesterol. Oatmeal is also a source of protein, calcium, iron, manganese, and B vitamins.

HOW TO SELECT AND STORE:

Cooking time and texture are the only differences among the varieties of oats used for oatmeal. Chewy steel-cut oats are whole oats sliced into thick pieces. Old-fashioned oats are steamed and flattened. Quick oats are cut into smaller pieces before being rolled. Instant oatmeal may have added sodium, and flavored versions have added sugar. Store in a dark, dry location in a well-sealed container for up to a year.

TIPS:

When preparing oatmeal on the stovetop, cooking time depends on the type of oats used. Steel-cut oats take about 20 minutes to cook on the stovetop. Old-fashioned oats, sometimes called "rolled oats," take about 5 minutes to cook. Quick oats cook in about a minute. Instant oatmeal is precooked so it takes only boiling water to reconstitute them. Try topping your oatmeal with fruit and nuts.

NUTRIENTS PER SERVING:

Oatmeal, ½ cup cooked
Calories: 83
Protein: 3g
Total fat: 2g
Saturated fat: 0g
Cholesterol: 0mg
Carbohydrate: 14g
Dietary fiber: 2g
Sodium: 5mg
Potassium: 80mg
Calcium: 11mg
Iron: 1.1mg
Magnesium: 32mg
Manganese: 0.7mg
Niacin: 0.3mg
Folate: 7mcg

CRANBERRY-ORANGE OATMEAL

3½ cups water

2 cups quick oats

¼ teaspoon salt

½ cup dried cranberries

1 large Gala apple, finely chopped

½ teaspoon grated orange peel

½ cup orange juice

¼ cup pecan pieces, toasted (see Tip)

⅓ cup sugar substitute

1 tablespoon ground cinnamon

1 teaspoon vanilla

1 tablespoon diet margarine

1. In a large saucepan, combine water, oats, salt, and cranberries. Cook according to directions on oatmeal container. Add apple, orange peel, juice, pecans, sugar substitute, cinnamon, vanilla, and margarine. Stir to combine.

NUTRIENTS PER SERVING:

Calories: 241
Calories from fat: 26%
Protein: 6g
Total fat: 7g
Saturated fat: <1g
Cholesterol: 0mg
Carbohydrate: 42g
Dietary fiber: 6g
Sodium: 147mg
Dietary exchanges:
2½ Starch, 1½ Fat

2. Cover. Let stand 5 minutes before serving.

Makes about 5 (1-cup) servings

Tip: To toast pecans, place in medium nonstick skillet over medium heat. Cook and stir about 3 minutes or until pecans begin to brown. Transfer immediately to a plate.

OLIVE OIL

NUTRIENTS PER SERVING:

Olive oil, 1 tablespoon
Calories: 119
Protein: 0g
Total fat: 13.5g
Saturated fat: 2g
Monounsaturated fat: 10g
Cholesterol: 0mg
Carbohydrate: 0g
Dietary fiber: 0g
Sodium: 0mg
Vitamin E: 1.9mg
Iron: 0.1mg

Olive oil should be a staple in your pantry. It's rich in heart-healthy fats, which are important for the many people with diabetes who also have heart disease.

BENEFITS:

Like all oils, olive oil contains a mix of saturated and unsaturated fats. Olive oil contains about 75 percent monounsaturated fat—making it one of the lowest of all oils in saturated fat, which raises levels of "bad" LDL cholesterol. Its high monounsaturated fat content has been shown to not only lower LDL levels when it replaces saturated fat in the diet, but to help raise levels of "good" HDL cholesterol. In addition, extra virgin and virgin olive oils are rich in polyphenols, antioxidants with strong heart-protective, anti-inflammatory action.

HOW TO SELECT AND STORE:

All types of olive oil contain the same calories and fat, but differ in color, flavor, and antioxidant content. Extra virgin and virgin olive oils have a greenish tint and are from the first and second pressing of the olives. Extra virgin olive oil is favored for its delicate flavor. Regular and light olive oils are more processed and lighter in color and flavor. Look for oils sold in dark tinted bottles, which protect the oil from going rancid via oxidation caused by exposure to light. Store olive oil in a cool area and use within a few months get the most from its antioxidants.

TIPS:

Due to its vast benefits, olive oil should be used in place of artery-clogging butter and margarine when cooking. Be careful when substituting olive oil in baking, as it will not work the same as butter or margarine.

ONIONS

Along with garlic, shallots, and leeks, onions are a member of the allium family and share many of the same health benefits, too. Onions can be used as a low-calorie flavorful ingredient in many dishes.

BENEFITS:

Onions contain the mineral chromium, which plays a crucial role for people with diabetes by enhancing insulin's ability to lower blood sugar levels. Like their garlic cousins, onions help to lower blood cholesterol levels and reduce blood clotting. Onions contain phytonutrients that fight inflammation and improve the integrity of blood vessels. And green onions provide vitamin A, which is essential for eye and skin health.

HOW TO SELECT AND STORE:

Onions can be found in various shapes and colors. Choose firm, dry onions with shiny, tissue-thin skins. Avoid those that are discolored or have wet spots. Onions keep three to four weeks in a dry, dark, cool location. Do not store them near potatoes, which give off a gas that causes onions to decay.

Look for green onions with crisp, not wilted, tops. Refrigerate green onions in an open plastic bag in the crisper drawer of the refrigerator.

NUTRIENTS PER SERVING:
Onions (white), ½ cup raw
Calories: 32
Protein: 1g
Total fat: 0g
Saturated fat: 0g
Cholesterol: 0mg
Carbohydrate: 8g
Dietary fiber: 1.5g
Sodium: 0mg
Potassium: 115mg
Calcium: 18mg
Iron: 0.2mg
Chromium: 12mcg
Vitamin C: 6mg
Folate: 15mcg

TIPS:

To minimize tears, slice onions under running water or chill before cutting. Sweet red and green onions are ideal raw. Other onions are best cooked to mellow their flavor. Sauté onions in a nonstick skillet with a small amount of oil or broth. When using green onions, be sure to trim roots and remove the outer layer before chopping.

ORANGES

In addition to providing insoluble fiber to help with blood sugar control, oranges pack nutrients that battle diabetes complications. Plus, their sweet, tart flavor makes them wonderful substitutes for high-calorie snacks and desserts.

BENEFITS:

This juicy fruit is best known for its vitamin C. One orange provides 130 percent of the daily requirement for vitamin C, which helps control infections, maintain healthy teeth and gums, and protect small blood vessels. As an antioxidant, vitamin C works with folate and potassium found to slow the development of coronary heart disease. Vitamin C and the phytochemical beta-carotene support eye health and lower the risk of sight-stealing cataracts.

HOW TO SELECT AND STORE:

Oranges are one of the few fruits abundant in winter. California navels are popular for eating on their own. The Valencias, produced in Florida, are the premier juice-producers. Mandarin oranges are small and sweet with thin skins and easily sectioned segments and are also available canned. Select firm fruit heavy for its size. Green color and blemishes are fine. Refrigerated, most varieties, except mandarins, will keep for two weeks. Orange juice is available fresh squeezed or from concentrate. Just be sure it has no added sugar.

NUTRIENTS PER SERVING:

Orange (navel), 1 medium
Calories: 69
Protein: 1g
Total fat: 0g
Saturated fat: 0g
Cholesterol: 0mg
Carbohydrate: 18g
Dietary fiber: 3g
Sodium: 0mg
Potassium: 230mg
Calcium: 60mg
Iron: 0.2mg
Vitamin A: 346 IU
Vitamin C: 83mg
Folate: 48mcg

TIPS:

For fruit salads or eating out of hand, choose seedless oranges. Top your favorite spinach salad with some orange segments. Use fresh orange juice to make marinades or nonfat sauces and dressings.

OREGANO

Skip harmful seasonings and sauces and sprinkle food with oregano to impart wonderful flavor. Of all the herbs, oregano has one of the highest antioxidant levels.

BENEFITS:

Beyond its role as a healthy flavor enhancer, oregano carries antioxidant nutrients that may give it even greater disease-fighting potential. Research into oregano's possible benefits is only in preliminary stages but suggests the herb may help with blood-sugar control and have positive effects on heart health and the integrity of blood vessels. Additionally, the lutein and zeaxanthin found in oregano may help prevent cataracts and certain other eye diseases.

HOW TO SELECT AND STORE:

Fresh oregano is often available in supermarkets. Choose bright green, fresh-looking bunches with no sign of wilting or yellowing. Refrigerate in a plastic bag for up to three days. Dried oregano is available in both crumbled and ground forms. It should be stored in a cool, dark place. Use dried oregano within six months.

TIPS:

Oregano has an aromatic scent and robust taste. It goes extremely well with tomato-based dishes, such as marinara sauce, tomato soup, and pizza. It also enhances cheese and egg dishes. Oregano can be combined with other herbs and garlic to create a rub marinade for meats. Fresh oregano is best used at the end of cooking or sprinkled on foods just before eating, whereas dried oregano can be added during cooking.

NUTRIENTS PER SERVING:

Oregano, 1 teaspoon dried
Calories: 3
Protein: 0g
Total fat: 0g
Saturated fat: 0g
Cholesterol: 0mg
Carbohydrate: <1g
Dietary fiber: 0.5g
Sodium: 0mg
Potassium: 13mg
Calcium: 16mg
Iron: 0.4mg
Vitamin A: 17 IU
Folate: 2mcg

PAPAYA

Tropical papaya is an amazing fruit that can weigh up to 20 pounds and is used both green and ripe. When ripe, its golden flesh has a buttery consistency and a sweet, musky taste.

BENEFITS:

Papayas are bursting with vitamins A and C, antioxidants that help reduce heart disease and cancer risks. The generous dose of C also fortifies your body's wound-healing ability and helps keep your immune system in shape. Papayas also provide plenty of potassium, an essential mineral that helps keep blood pressure in a healthy range. The fiber in papayas is mostly soluble, so it helps lower blood cholesterol.

HOW TO SELECT AND STORE:

The most commonly available papayas are grown in Hawaii; they are pear-shaped and weigh about a pound. Mexican papayas are much larger, longer, and heavier. Look for papayas that have yellow to reddish-orange skin and yield slightly to pressure. If slightly green, leave them at room temperature to ripen for a few days. Refrigerate and use ripe fruit as soon as possible. Unripe, green papayas are usually cooked as a vegetable.

NUTRIENTS PER SERVING:

Papaya, ½ medium raw
Calories: 68
Protein: 1g
Total fat: 0g
Saturated fat: 0g
Cholesterol: 0mg
Carbohydrate: 17g
Dietary fiber: 3g
Sodium: 15mg
Potassium: 285mg
Calcium: 31mg
Iron: 0.4mg
Vitamin A: 1,492 IU
Vitamin C: 96mg
Folate: 58mcg

TIPS:

Wash papayas and slice them lengthwise before scooping out the seeds. The peppery seeds are edible, but bitter. Try papaya as a breakfast treat with a squeeze of lime juice and a pinch of crushed red pepper. It's an excellent addition to salsas and makes an attractive, edible container for fruit salads.

PARSLEY

This herb is more than a garnish. Parsley is rich in beneficial nutrients for people with diabetes.

BENEFITS:

Folk medicine suggests parsley as a treatment for diabetes, and animal studies have shown it has some ability to lower blood sugar, although further research is needed. Parsley does provide nutrients that can help ward off diabetes-related problems. It's rich in beta-carotene and vitamin C as well as flavonoids—all of which help protect against diabetes-related complications, including inflammation and damage to blood vessels, which can lead to heart attacks, strokes, and vision loss.

HOW TO SELECT AND STORE:

Although there are several varieties, the most common forms of fresh parsley are curly-leaf and Italian flat-leaf. Choose parsley with bright green leaves and no wilting or yellowing. Store a bunch of parsley in a plastic bag in the refrigerator. Or you can place the stems in a cup of water, cover the tops loosely with plastic wrap, and refrigerate for up to a week. Dried parsley is available in the spice section.

TIPS:

Fresh parsley should be rinsed well and patted dry. The leaves are often removed for chopping, but parts of the stem can also be used. Fresh parsley can be used in salads. The traditional Middle Eastern tabbouleh salad contains curly-leaf parsley. Italian flat-leaf parsley is best used in cooked dishes, including soups, stews, stuffing, sauces, vegetable dishes, eggs, savory pies, and casseroles. It can be cooked into a dish or sprinkled on top before serving.

PASTA

This comfort food is no longer banned from a diabetic diet. Whole wheat and whole grain pastas are a tasty way to enjoy this favorite fare without worrying about your blood sugar.

BENEFITS:

Whole grain and whole wheat pastas are naturally rich in fiber, which slows the absorption of sugar, and in minerals, such as magnesium, that increase the body's sensitivity to insulin. This makes whole wheat or whole grain pasta a must, as these beneficial ingredients are typically lost or significantly reduced when grains are refined. Newer varieties of healthy pastas, including products with added fiber, are especially helpful for diabetic diets.

HOW TO SELECT AND STORE:

To simplify your pasta choices, look for products labeled as whole wheat or whole grain. Whole wheat pasta is darker and tends to have a chewier texture than white. Whole grain pasta is made with a mix of nutrient-rich ingredients, including legumes, oats, barley, flax, and egg whites. Whole wheat and whole grain pastas cook about the same as white. Follow package instructions to be sure. Dried pasta will keep in your cupboard for several months.

TIPS:

Pasta is best cooked until al dente—tender yet chewy. Drain immediately and do not rinse. To prevent sticking, immediately toss with a low-fat vegetable sauce or olive oil. Toss some whole wheat pasta with your favorite beans and vegetables, drizzle with olive oil, and add a squeeze of lemon and some fresh herbs.

NUTRIENTS PER SERVING:

Pasta (whole wheat), ½ cup cooked

Calories: 87
Protein: 3.5g
Total fat: 0g
Saturated fat: 0g
Cholesterol: 0mg
Carbohydrate: 19g
Dietary fiber: 3g
Sodium: 0mg
Potassium: 30mg
Calcium: 10mg
Iron: 0.7mg
Vitamin A: 2 IU
Folate: 4mcg

PEACHES

In China, the peach symbolizes a long life. Perhaps that's because fresh peaches are a good source of an array of nutrients.

BENEFITS:

Fresh peaches are a low-calorie source of beta-carotene and vitamin C—antioxidant nutrients that researchers believe may help prevent complications of diabetes, such as nerve damage and eye disease. Peaches also supply soluble fiber that helps prevent spikes in blood sugar levels.

HOW TO SELECT AND STORE:

Peaches are at their best in late summer. A fresh peach's velvety skin can range from golden-red to creamy-pink with flesh that is bright orange to creamy-white. Look for fragrant fruit that gives slightly to pressure. Be cautious of soft spots, as peaches bruise easily. Place peaches in a paper bag with an apple to speed up the ripening process. Once ripe, they will last in the refrigerator for up to five days. When fresh peaches aren't available, try frozen, canned, or dried peaches. To keep calories low, look for canned peaches in water or juice, and frozen or dried peaches without added sugar.

NUTRIENTS PER SERVING:
Peach, 1 medium raw
Calories: 58
Protein: 1g
Total fat: 0g
Saturated fat: 0g
Cholesterol: 0mg
Carbohydrate: 14g
Dietary fiber: 2g
Sodium: 0mg
Potassium: 285mg
Calcium: 9mg
Iron: 0.4mg
Vitamin A: 489 IU
Vitamin C: 10mg
Folate: 6mcg

TIPS:

Rinse fresh peaches and enjoy with the peel for more fiber. Peaches can be enjoyed as a light snack, in fruit salads, salsas, and smoothies. They can be mixed with low-fat cottage cheese for a light breakfast. For a fun summer meal, try grilling or broiling fresh peach halves on a kabob with your favorite meat or poultry. Just season peaches with a touch of cinnamon or nutmeg to get a sweet, smoky flavor.

PEANUT BUTTER

Peanut butter is rich in protein and provides long-lasting energy and essential heart-protective nutrients with little effect on blood sugar.

BENEFITS:

The combination of protein, fiber, and fat in peanut butter means it digests more slowly and provides fuel over time without causing blood sugar spikes. Peanut butter is rich in monounsaturated fats, which help lower bad LDL cholesterol; niacin, which helps raise good HDL cholesterol levels; and potassium for blood pressure control. Peanut butter contains a high amount of magnesium, a mineral that is often found in low levels in people with diabetes.

HOW TO SELECT AND STORE:

Peanut butter is available in many varieties. Natural peanut butter is unprocessed and the oil may separate out. Simply stir to combine and refrigerate for up to six months. Make your own peanut butter with shelled peanuts in the food processor. Homemade peanut butter keeps about three months in the refrigerator. When buying from the store, look for peanut butters with little or no added sugar.

TIPS:

Rather than your typical PB&J, try a peanut butter and banana or peanut butter and honey sandwich. Peanut butter has many uses besides sandwiches. Enjoy it for a snack spread on apple wedges, pears, or crackers. Pay attention to portions—a little peanut butter goes a long way.

NUTRIENTS PER SERVING:

Peanut butter, 2 tablespoons unsalted (low sodium)

Calories: 188
Protein: 8g
Total fat: 16g
Saturated fat: 3g
Monounsaturated fat: 8g
Polyunsaturated fat: 4g
Cholesterol: 0mg
Carbohydrate: 6g
Dietary fiber: 2g
Sodium: 5mg
Potassium: 208mg
Magnesium: 49mg
Phosphorus: 115mg
Calcium: 14mg
Iron: 1mg
Folate: 41mcg
Niacin: 4mg
Vitamin B$_6$: 0.2mg
Vitamin E: 3mg

CHOCOLATE PEANUT BUTTER ICE CREAM SANDWICHES

2 tablespoons creamy peanut butter

8 chocolate wafer cookies

⅓ cup no-sugar-added vanilla ice cream, softened

NUTRIENTS PER SERVING:

1 sandwich
Calories: 129
Calories from fat: 49%
Total fat: 7g
Saturated fat: 3g
Cholesterol: 4mg
Sodium: 124mg
Carbohydrate: 15g
Dietary fiber: 1g
Protein: 4g
Dietary exchanges:
1 Starch, 1 Fat

1. Spread peanut butter evenly over flat sides of all cookies.

2. Spoon ice cream over peanut butter on 4 cookies. Top with remaining 4 cookies, peanut butter sides down. Press down lightly to force ice cream to edges of sandwiches.

3. Wrap each sandwich tightly in foil. Freeze at least 2 hours or up to 5 days.

Makes 4 servings

PEARS

The juicy flavor and crisp bite of pears make them a delightful snack. They are filled with fiber to help keep blood sugar levels intact.

BENEFITS:

You can't pick a fruit that outpaces pears in fiber. Pears' soluble fiber helps keep blood sugar in a more desirable range, likely decreasing the risk of diabetes-related complications. It also helps protect the more fragile diabetic heart and blood vessels by decreasing the bad LDL cholesterol. Pears provide heart-healthy potassium, vitamin C, and folate, too. While more research is needed, recent studies indicate that certain flavonoids contained in pears can help improve insulin sensitivity.

NUTRIENTS PER SERVING:

Pear, 1 medium raw
Calories: 103
Protein: 1g
Total fat: 0g
Saturated fat: 0g
Cholesterol: 0mg
Carbohydrate: 28g
Dietary fiber: 5.5g
Sodium: 0mg
Potassium: 210mg
Calcium: 16mg
Iron: 0.3mg
Vitamin A: 41 IU
Vitamin C: 8mg
Folate: 12mcg

HOW TO SELECT AND STORE:

The juicy fresh Bartletts are the most common variety and are also available canned. The red and green Anjous, which are firmer and not quite as sweet, are all-purpose pears. So are the Boscs, which have elongated necks and unusual dull-russet coloring. Bosc pears are crunchy, while Comice pears are sweetest. Pears ripen from the inside out, so buy them firm but not rock hard. Ripen them on the counter or in a paper bag, but don't pile them up or they'll bruise. Canned pears have more calories when packed in syrup and less fiber without their skins. Choose cloudy pear juice over clear pear juice.

TIPS:

To get a pear's full nutritional value, eat the skin. Firm pears do well in salads or for cooking. Ripe pears are great mixed with nonfat yogurt and cereal. Bartlett and Bosc pears are good for cooking.

PECANS

Whether you call them "pee-canz" or "pa-kawnz," these elegant, versatile, rich-tasting nuts offer nutrients that can help protect you from diabetes-related damage.

BENEFITS:

Pecans contain a ton of nutrients that can help protect you from certain diabetes-related conditions, especially heart disease. Studies have shown that including just a few ounces of pecans daily in a heart-healthy diet can reduce damaging triglyceride and LDL cholesterol levels while increasing protective HDL cholesterol levels. Pecans contain vitamin E, which helps prevent free-radical damage to the heart and blood vessels, as well as minerals potassium, calcium, and magnesium, which help lower blood pressure. One serving, about 19 pecans, provides about 10 percent of the daily requirement of fiber, which is also associated with a lower risk of heart disease.

NUTRIENTS PER SERVING:

Pecans, 1 ounce dry roasted without salt
Calories: 201
Protein: 3g
Total fat: 21g
Saturated fat: 2g
Cholesterol: 0mg
Carbohydrate: 4g
Dietary fiber: 2.5g
Sodium: 0mg
Potassium: 120mg
Phosphorus: 83mg
Calcium: 20mg
Iron: 0.8mg
Zinc: 1.4mg
Magnesium: 37mg
Vitamin A: 40 IU

HOW TO SELECT AND STORE:

Shelled pecans are available as halves, chips, or ground and may be raw, dry roasted or oil roasted, salted or unsalted. Unsalted raw pecans are usually used in recipes, while roasted varieties are best for snacking. Choose unsalted dry roasted pecans. Refrigerated, shelled pecans will keep up to nine months. Unshelled pecans will keep for three to six months in a cool, dry place.

TIPS:

Use pecans to top salads, vegetables, and cereal. They add flavor and crunch to cookies, muffins, and other baked goods. Try breading chicken or fish with ground pecans for a lower-carbohydrate dinner.

PINEAPPLE

Pineapple gets high scores for its exceptionally sweet and tart taste and health-protective nutrients. It satisfies your sweet tooth, too.

BENEFITS:

Pineapple provides more than a third of the daily recommended allowance of vitamin C, which helps with immune health. This is important for people with diabetes because they a have a higher risk of infection. Vitamin C is also a powerful antioxidant that helps protect against diabetes-related heart disease. Pineapple offers heart-protective folate and potassium, as well, which are needed for healthy blood pressure.

HOW TO SELECT AND STORE:

When choosing pineapple, let your nose be your guide. A ripe pineapple gives off a sweet aroma from its base. Color is not a reliable indicator; ripe pineapples vary in color by variety. Choose a large pineapple that feels heavy for its size. A ripe pineapple yields slightly when pressed. Once a pineapple is picked, it will not ripen further. Canned pineapple is available; select varieties packed in juice or water, not syrup.

NUTRIENTS PER SERVING:

Pineapple, ½ cup raw
Calories: 41
Protein: 1g
Total fat: 0g
Saturated fat: 0g
Cholesterol: 0mg
Carbohydrate: 11g
Dietary fiber: 1g
Sodium: 0mg
Potassium: 90mg
Calcium: 11mg
Iron: 0.2mg
Manganese: 0.8mg
Vitamin C: 39mg
Folate: 15mcg

TIPS:

Preparing a pineapple is not as scary it looks. Cut off the bottom and top, then peel the outside using a sharp knife. Remove any remaining "eyes." Cut into quarters and remove the core from each quarter and cut into slices. Add pineapple to a fruit smoothie, fruit salad, or on top low-fat yogurt. Make fruit kabobs with pineapple for a unique dessert. Pineapple works well when grilled. Try it alone for dessert or on a kabob with your favorite meat.

PISTACHIOS

Compared to other popular nuts, pistachios are among the highest in protein and fiber and also one of the lowest in calories and fat.

BENEFITS:

Pistachios are useful for people with diabetes who also have heart disease. These yummy green nuts are full of phytosterols, natural compounds that compete with cholesterol for absorption by the body, helping reduce blood cholesterol levels. Pistachios are rich in heart-healthy monounsaturated fats. They provide a hefty amount of resveratrol, a phytonutrient (also found in wine) that may play a role in fighting heart disease and cancer. Additionally, pistachios offer potassium, magnesium, copper, vitamin B_6, and vitamin E.

HOW TO SELECT AND STORE:

Pistachios are increasingly available shelled but are more expensive than unshelled forms. They are available either raw or roasted, and salted or unsalted. Unshelled pistachios should be partly opened, which not only makes it easier to remove the nut, but also indicates that the nut is mature and ready to be eaten. Store pistachios in an airtight container in the refrigerator or freezer for up to one year.

NUTRIENTS PER SERVING:

Pistachios, 1 ounce dry roasted without salt

Calories: 161
Protein: 6g
Total fat: 13g
Saturated fat: 1.5g
Cholesterol: 0mg
Carbohydrate: 8g
Dietary fiber: 3g
Sodium: 0mg
Potassium: 285mg
Calcium: 30mg
Iron: 1.1mg
Vitamin A: 73 IU
Vitamin C: 1mg
Folate: 14mcg
Magnesium: 31mg
Vitamin E: 0.7mg

TIPS:

Pistachios can be toasted and added to vegetable or rice dishes. Sprinkle a handful of chopped pistachios on breakfast cereal or salads for an extra crunch. Swap them out with walnuts that are traditionally used in baking. Incorporate them into muffins, cakes, or cookies.

PLUMS

You can't go wrong with this juicy fruit. Considering their small size, plums provide quite a hefty amount of nutrients.

BENEFITS:

Plums provide minimal calories and a generous dose of vitamins A and C, potassium and fiber, nutrients that provide protection against diabetes-related complications, including damage to the blood vessel. Dried plums, or prunes, are especially beneficial for diabetes, as they're a concentrated source of soluble fiber, which helps increase insulin sensitivity and helps to stabilize blood sugar levels.

HOW TO SELECT AND STORE:

Plums are a summer fruit with a long season from May through October. Some plums cling to their pits while others have "free" stones (pits). Plum skins come in a rainbow of colors: red, purple, black, green, blue, and even yellow. The flesh can be yellow, orange, green, or red. Look for plump plums with a bright or deep color. If it yields to gentle pressure, it's ripe. Once slightly soft, plums should be eaten or refrigerated soon after.

TIPS:

Like many fruits, plums taste sweetest at room temperature. Plums can be added to fruit salads, baked goods, compotes, puddings, or meat dishes. They can also be made into butters, jams, purees, or sauces. Pureed dried plums (prunes) make a fabulous fat substitute in recipes for quick breads, muffins, and other baked goods. Not only do they substantially reduce calories, they also boost their nutrition content.

NUTRIENTS PER SERVING:

Plum, 1 medium raw
Calories: 30
Protein: <1g
Total fat: 0g
Saturated fat: 0g
Cholesterol: 0mg
Carbohydrate: 7g
Dietary fiber: 1g
Sodium: 0mg
Potassium: 105mg
Calcium: 4mg
Iron: 0.1mg
Vitamin A: 228 IU
Vitamin C: 6mg
Folate: 3mcg

POMEGRANATE

The jewel-like interior of a pomegranate, its sparkling little seeds, and its juice are loaded with nutrients.

BENEFITS:

Don't be intimidated by their large size—pomegranates are great for any diet because the juicy seeds are full of fiber yet low in calories. Pomegranate juice is nutritious as well, but lacks any fiber. Both the seeds and the juice are rich in disease-fighting antioxidants that may help reduce artery-clogging plaque by lowering levels of LDL (bad) cholesterol. Pomegranates offer up plenty of potassium, a mineral that plays an important role in blood pressure control.

HOW TO SELECT AND STORE:

Fresh pomegranates are at their best in late fall and early winter. Choose fresh pomegranates with a bright, deep red color and un-blemished skin that feel heavy for their size. Refrigerate for up to two months or store in a cool, dark place for up to a month. Once cut, seeds can be refrigerated for about three days or frozen. Pomegranate juice is available in bottles, as concentrate, or in combination with other juices.

TIPS:

Eating a fresh pomegranate is messy business and the juice stains, so dress accordingly. Cut the pomegranate in half and pry out the seeds, removing the light-colored membrane. For easier removal, soak cut sections of pomegranate in a bowl of water to loosen the seeds; the membrane will float to the top. Pomegranate seeds make a gorgeous garnish. Enjoy the crunchy seeds on their own, or use them to top salads or yogurt. Pomegranate juice can be used in marinades and sauces.

NUTRIENTS PER SERVING:

Pomegranate, ½ cup raw
Calories: 72
Protein: 1g
Total fat: 1g
Saturated fat: 0g
Cholesterol: 0mg
Carbohydrate: 16g
Dietary fiber: 3.5g
Sodium: 0mg
Potassium: 205mg
Calcium: 9mg
Iron: 0.3mg
Vitamin C: 9mg
Folate: 33mcg

BREAKFAST POM SMOOTHIE

1 small ripe banana

¾ cup pomegranate juice

½ cup mixed berries

⅓ to ½ cup soymilk or milk

NUTRIENTS PER SERVING:

Calories: 253
Protein: 3g
Total fat: 1g
Saturated fat: 1g
Cholesterol: 0mg
Carbohydrate: 59g
Dietary fiber: 6g
Sodium: 35mg
Dietary exchanges: 1 Starch, 3 Fruit

1. Combine banana and berries in blender; process until smooth.

2. Add juice and soymilk; process until smooth. Serve immediately.

Makes 1 (1½-cup) serving

Variations: Substitute pomegranate-blueberry juice or any other pomegranate juice blend for the pomegranate juice. You can also substitute yogurt for the soymilk.

POPCORN

Popcorn is a surprising snack food that people with diabetes can indulge in. Like other whole grain sources of carbohydrate, air-popped and unprocessed popcorn is a good source of fiber and nutrients.

BENEFITS:

Plain popcorn is a delicious snack that's naturally low in calories and fat. Plus, you can have a large volume for a small amount of calories. Because it's made from corn, a whole grain, popcorn doesn't impact blood sugar levels as much as many other snack foods. Popcorn also has a lower glycemic load than raisins, rice cakes, or potato chips. Air-popped popcorn without added butter or oil is a good source of potassium, magnesium, and phosphorus.

HOW TO SELECT AND STORE:

Popcorn is available in the snack food aisle in various flavors and forms. Buy popcorn kernels to pop yourself on the stovetop or in an air popper, or look for low-fat microwave popcorn. Avoid the heavily salted and buttery varieties of popcorn. Choose low-fat varieties of popcorn without added fats, sugars, and salts.

TIPS:

Rather than dousing your popcorn in butter and salt, experiment with healthier alternatives that add flavor, not guilt. Try adding garlic powder rather than salt. If you love kettle corn, try sprinkling ground cinnamon and a sugar substitute for a sweet snack.

NUTRIENTS PER SERVING:

Popcorn, 2 cups air-popped without added butter or oil

Calories: 62
Protein: 2g
Total fat: 1g
Saturated fat: 0g
Cholesterol: 0mg
Carbohydrate: 12g
Dietary fiber: 2g
Calcium: 1mg
Potassium: 53mg
Sodium: 1mg
Magnesium: 23mg
Phosphorus: 57mg

CINNAMON CARAMEL CORN

8 cups air-popped popcorn (about ⅓ cup kernels)
2 tablespoons honey
4 teaspoons butter
¼ teaspoon ground cinnamon

1. Preheat oven to 350°F. Spray jelly-roll pan with nonstick cooking spray. Place popcorn in large bowl.

2. Cook and stir honey, butter, and cinnamon in small saucepan over low heat until butter is melted and mixture is smooth; immediately pour over popcorn. Toss to coat evenly. Pour onto prepared pan; bake 12 to 14 minutes or until coating is golden brown and appears crackled, stirring twice during baking time.

3. Let cool on pan 5 minutes. (As popcorn cools, coating becomes crisp. If not crisp enough, or if popcorn softens upon standing, return to oven and heat 5 to 8 minutes.) Cool completely. Store in airtight container.

Makes 4 servings

NUTRIENTS PER SERVING:

Caramel corn, 2 cups
Calories: 117
Calories from fat: 29%
Protein: 2g
Total fat: 4g
Saturated fat: 1g
Cholesterol: 0mg
Carbohydrate: 19g
Dietary fiber: 1g
Sodium: 45mg
Dietary exchanges:
1 Starch, 1 Fat

Cajun Popcorn: Preheat oven and prepare jelly-roll pan as directed above. Combine 7 teaspoons honey, 4 teaspoons butter, and 1 teaspoon Cajun or Creole seasoning in a small saucepan. Proceed with recipe as directed above.

Italian Popcorn: Spray 8 cups of air-popped popcorn with fat-free butter-flavored spray to coat. Sprinkle with 2 tablespoons finely grated Parmesan cheese, ⅛ teaspoon black pepper, and ½ teaspoon dried oregano; toss to coat.

PORK TENDERLOIN

Pork tenderloin is lean and rich in plenty of nutrients, making it a great substitute for the poultry you may be getting sick of.

BENEFITS:

Pork tenderloin is comparable to skinless chicken breast in calories, total fat, and saturated fat. It's lower in cholesterol, so it's a good fit for a heart-healthy diabetes diet. Its high quality protein leaves you feeling satisfied, which will help in any weight-loss efforts. Pork tenderloin also provides more than 20 percent of your daily requirements for many B vitamins, including thiamin, niacin, riboflavin, vitamin B_6, and the mineral phosphorus. This is significant since the body needs B vitamins to turn food into energy.

NUTRIENTS PER SERVING:

Pork tenderloin, 3 ounces roasted

Calories: 125
Protein: 22g
Total fat: 3.5g
Saturated fat: 1g
Cholesterol: 62mg
Carbohydrate: <1g
Dietary fiber: 0g
Sodium: 50mg
Potassium: 355mg
Thiamin: 0.8mg
Riboflavin: 0.3mg
Niacin: 6.3mg
Vitamin B_6: 0.6mg
Phosphorus: 225mg

HOW TO SELECT AND STORE:

Pork tenderloin is long and thin and easy to find in the supermarket's fresh meat section. About 4 ounces raw will yield a 3-ounce cooked serving. Prepackaged fresh pork tenderloin can be stored in the refrigerator for up to four days. Well-wrapped, it can be stored in the freezer for up to six months.

TIPS:

Pork tenderloin makes an elegant entrée for a dinner party but also can easily be roasted or grilled for a quick meal. It has a mild flavor, so it's best when prepared with an added spice rub, marinade, stuffing, or flavorful sauce. To keep the tenderloin juicy, be careful not to overcook it. A meat thermometer inserted into the thickest part of the meat should reach a temperature of 160°F for medium doneness.

POTATOES

While potatoes may seem unhealthy, they aren't. They are packed with nutrients that can actually assist in controlling the disease.

BENEFITS:

Potatoes are packed with heart-protective, immune-boosting vitamin C and blood-pressure-lowering potassium. They're rather filling yet free of fat and cholesterol. While they are high in carbohydrates, you can make them more diabetes friendly by leaving the peel on. Eating the potato with its skin on provides a richer dose of fiber to help slow digestion and limit the rise in blood sugar. Because some of the fiber is soluble, it also helps lower blood cholesterol.

HOW TO SELECT AND STORE:

There are more than hundred varieties of potatoes. Russets are best for baking while new potatoes (those harvested before maturity and much smaller) are best-suited for boiling. Choose potatoes that are firm with no soft or dark spots. Store in a dry, cool, dark, ventilated location, away from onions. Mature potatoes keep for several weeks. New potatoes keep only one week.

NUTRIENTS PER SERVING:

Potato, 1 medium baked
Calories: 161
Protein: 4g
Total fat: 0g
Saturated fat: 0g
Cholesterol: 0mg
Carbohydrate: 37g
Dietary fiber: 4g
Sodium: 15mg
Potassium: 925mg
Calcium: 26mg
Iron: 1.9mg
Vitamin A: 17 IU
Vitamin C: 17mg
Folate: 48mcg

TIPS:

Just before cooking, scrub potatoes well with a vegetable brush and cut out sprout buds and bad spots. Baking a potato takes an hour in the oven but only five minutes in the microwave. Try a healthy version of a loaded baked potato: Top with nonfat yogurt and sprinkle with chopped dill or scallions. For a French fry fix, toss thin-cut potatoes with olive oil and season with salt and pepper; roast in a 400°F oven for about 30 minutes.

Pumpkin Seeds

Pumpkin seeds, or pepitas, are rich in protein, fiber, and unsaturated fats, making them a great fit for a diabetic diet.

BENEFITS:

Pumpkin seeds can help stabilize blood sugar levels. The fat they contain is mostly monounsaturated and omega-3 polyunsaturated, which help lower total and "bad" LDL cholesterol and raise beneficial HDL cholesterol. A diet rich in these fats is associated with a lower risk of coronary heart disease, a common diabetes-related condition. Pumpkin seeds also offer potassium and magnesium, which help lower blood pressure.

HOW TO SELECT AND STORE:

Pumpkin seeds can be purchased with or without the white hull, roasted or raw, and with or without salt. Dry roasted pumpkin seeds without salt are healthiest. The pepitas are often sold roasted and salted in the Mexican food section but may also be available raw or unsalted. Pumpkin seeds will keep in an airtight container in a cool, dark place for several months.

NUTRIENTS PER SERVING:

Pumpkin seeds, 1 ounce dry roasted without salt
Calories: 63
Protein: 3g
Total fat: 3g
Saturated fat: 0.5g
Cholesterol: 0mg
Carbohydrate: 8g
Dietary fiber: 2.5g
Sodium: 0mg
Potassium: 130mg
Calcium: 8mg
Iron: 0.5mg
Vitamin A: 9 IU
Folate: 1mcg
Magnesium: 37mg
Vitamin E: 0mg

TIPS:

Whole pumpkin seeds are easy to prepare. Scoop them out of the pumpkin, wash them, and let them dry out. Bake them on a greased baking sheet at 250°F for about an hour or until crisp. Lightly salt them while warm, if desired. Enjoy them as a crunchy snack or add them with other nuts and dried fruits for a fun trail mix. Pepitas can be sprinkled on salads or baked into breads and cookies.

QUINOA

With more protein and fiber than most grains, quinoa makes a great guilt-free addition to a diabetic meal plan.

BENEFITS:

Quinoa contains fewer carbohydrates and more protein than rice and other grains, making it less likely to cause blood sugar spikes. Its protein content is similar to meat, so it's quite filling. Quinoa has the added benefit of heart-healthy unsaturated fats rather than the saturated fats found in meat and dairy. Quinoa is rich in phytonutrients that help protect against cardiovascular disease and other diabetes-related conditions. Its fiber, magnesium, and vitamin E may help improve insulin sensitivity.

NUTRIENTS PER SERVING:

Quinoa, ½ cup cooked
Calories: 111
Protein: 4g
Total fat: 2g
Saturated fat: 0g
Cholesterol: 0mg
Carbohydrate: 20g
Dietary fiber: 2.5g
Sodium: 6mg
Potassium: 160mg
Iron: 1.4mg
Zinc: 1mg
Magnesium: 59mg
Phosphorus: 141mg
Folate: 39mcg
Vitamin E: 0.6mg

HOW TO SELECT AND STORE:

Quinoa is available in many supermarkets near the rice and other grains. It has a tiny, beaded shape and may be red, black, or ivory-colored. Dry quinoa should be stored in a sealed container in a cool, dry place or in the refrigerator. Quinoa is also available ground into flour and in several forms of pasta.

TIPS:

Rinse quinoa before cooking in a fine-mesh sieve. Combine one part quinoa to one and a half parts water or broth in a medium or large saucepan. (It will expand to four times its original volume.) Bring to a simmer and reduce to low heat. Cover and cook for about 15 minutes; let stand 5 minutes and then fluff with a fork. Quinoa works well in soups, salads, side dishes, hot breakfast cereals, and even faux rice pudding.

RASPBERRIES

These sweet, juicy berries pack fabulous flavor and some serious punch when it comes to helping you fend off diabetes complications.

BENEFITS:

Raspberries are great for any diet; they are low in calories and provide a whopping 8 grams of fiber per cup. They're high in pectin, a soluble fiber that helps steady blood sugar levels as well as lower blood cholesterol, which is often elevated in people with diabetes. Among raspberries' phytonutrients are anthocyanins, which have been found to help reduce blood sugar after a carbohydrate-rich meal. Raspberries also contain an appreciable amount of vitamin C, an antioxidant that offers immune protection, which is helpful for people with diabetes who are at greater risk for infections.

HOW TO SELECT AND STORE:

Raspberries are fragile and should be handled carefully and eaten soon after purchasing. Look for brightly colored berries with no hulls attached. Avoid any that look shriveled or have visible mold. They should be plump, firm, well shaped, and packed in a shallow container. Frozen, unsweetened raspberries work well in smoothies and baked goods.

TIPS:

Rinse raspberries under cool water just before serving. Puree fresh or frozen raspberries to create a sweet and tart sauce to top a fruit salad. Add raspberries to yogurt for a healthy and tasty breakfast. If you're celebrating a special occasion, enjoy a glass of champagne with some chilled raspberries. Raspberries also make a colorful garnish.

NUTRIENTS PER SERVING:

Raspberries, ½ cup raw
Calories: 32
Protein: 1g
Total fat: 0g
Saturated fat: 0g
Cholesterol: 0mg
Carbohydrate: 7g
Dietary fiber: 4g
Sodium: 0mg
Potassium: 95mg
Calcium: 15mg
Iron: 0.4mg
Vitamin A: 20 IU
Vitamin C: 16mg
Folate: 13mcg

RYE BREAD

Move over, wheat! Their hearty flavor and numerous health benefits make rye foods worth including in your meal plan.

BENEFITS:

Like other whole grains, rye products are rich in fiber that helps keep blood sugar from skyrocketing following a meal. Compared to whole wheat bread, rye bread contains more iron and B vitamins. Rye bread has also been shown to trigger less of an insulin response, so blood sugar is less likely to plunge, too. And as an added bonus, rye bread keeps you feeling satisfied longer, making it easier to manage your appetite between meals.

HOW TO SELECT AND STORE:

Rye grains are generally ground into flour. Dark rye flour retains most of the bran and germ, so it has more fiber and nutrients than light rye flour. Store rye grains in an airtight container in a cool, dry, dark place, where they'll keep for several months. Rye bread is available in the bread section of the supermarket. Read labels carefully, as what is labeled "rye bread" is sometimes wheat bread with caramel coloring.

NUTRIENTS PER SERVING:

Rye bread, 1 slice
Calories: 83
Protein: 3g
Total fat: 1g
Saturated fat: 0g
Cholesterol: 0mg
Carbohydrate: 15g
Dietary fiber: 2g
Sodium: 211mg
Potassium: 53mg
Calcium: 23mg
Iron: 0.9mg
Thiamin: 0.14mg
Riboflavin: 0.1mg
Folate: 35mcg

TIPS:

Rye bread is more compact and dense than wheat bread, so it works well for toasting or for sandwiches. Rye bread pairs well with corned beef. For a tasty snack or appetizer, make Reuben bites. Bake party-size rye bread slices in a 400°F oven for 5 minutes. Spread fat-free Thousand Island dressing on the mini bread slices. Top with turkey pastrami and shredded reduced-fat Swiss cheese. Bake for another 5 minutes. Top with alfalfa sprouts and serve immediately.

SALMON

NUTRIENTS PER SERVING:

Salmon (wild Atlantic), 3 ounces roasted
Calories: 155
Protein: 22g
Total fat: 7g
Saturated fat: 1g
Cholesterol: 60mg
Carbohydrate: 0g
Dietary fiber: 0g
Sodium: 50mg
Potassium: 535mg
Calcium: 13mg
Iron: 0.9mg
Phosphorus: 218mg
Selenium: 40mcg
Niacin: 8.6mg

Whether enjoyed hot as a main dish, on top of a salad, or cold in a sandwich, salmon is rich in flavor and beneficial nutrients, making it a great alternative to the more typical whitefish.

BENEFITS:

Although salmon can be a fatty fish, most of the fat is omega-3s, healthy polyunsaturated fatty acids. Omega-3 fish oil helps protect against heart disease, a common diabetes complication, and improves the body's ability to respond to insulin. Omega-3s may also stimulate secretion of leptin, a hormone that helps regulate food intake, body weight, and metabolism. Because a diet that includes fatty fish is so consistently associated with a variety of health benefits, recent U.S. government guidelines recommend that all Americans eat fish twice a week.

HOW TO SELECT AND STORE:

Salmon is classified as either Pacific or Atlantic. There is only one species of Atlantic salmon, but there are five species of Pacific, including Chinook (king), sockeye (red), Coho (silver), pink, and chum. Some salmon are richer and fattier than others; but remember, it is heart-healthy fat. Look for fresh salmon with flesh that is firm to the touch. Whenever possible, choose wild rather than farm-raised salmon. Fresh salmon is available whole or in steak or fillet form. Salmon is also available frozen, canned, dried, or smoked.

TIPS:

Salmon can be grilled, baked, broiled, or steamed. It is naturally moist and tender and requires little seasoning, but a light sauce, such as teriyaki or honey mustard, complements the rich flavor.

SCALLOPS

In addition to their scrumptious taste, scallops have a variety of nutrients that can help promote cardiovascular health.

BENEFITS:

Scallops are a type of shellfish. This category of seafood includes any water-dwelling creature that wears its skeleton on the outside. All shellfish are lean, rich in nutrients, and high in protein. Weight for weight, they have more vitamin B_{12} than any other animal protein. Scallops provide heart-healthy omega-3s, and also offer magnesium and potassium, which helps lower blood pressure.

HOW TO SELECT AND STORE:

Because scallops are so perishable, they are typically shelled, washed, and frozen, or packed in ice as soon as they are caught. The season for fresh sea and bay scallops runs from October to March. Fresh calico scallops are available from December to May. Fresh scallops should have white, firm flesh with no browning. Frozen scallops are available year-round and should be solid and shiny. Fresh scallops will keep for a day or two in the refrigerator. Frozen scallops will last for a month or two.

TIPS:

Scallops don't need much cooking time. The flesh will be rubbery and tough if overcooked. Try sautéing scallops with mushrooms and scallions. Or serve scallops with a sauce made from fresh tarragon, white wine, and blood orange juice. Try adding scallops to your gazpacho.

NUTRIENTS PER SERVING:

Scallops, 3 ounces cooked without fat
Calories: 93
Protein: 18g
Total fat: 1g
Saturated fat: 0g
Cholesterol: 35mg
Carbohydrate: 2g
Dietary fiber: 0g
Sodium: 441mg
Calcium: 26mg
Magnesium: 59mg
Potassium: 340mg
Phosphorus: 231mg
Vitamin B$_{12}$: 1.5mcg
Selenium: 23mcg
Zinc: 1mg

SCALLIONED SCALLOPS

¼ cup all-purpose flour
½ teaspoon dried thyme
½ teaspoon paprika
¼ teaspoon ground red pepper
1 pound scallops, rinsed and patted dry
2 teaspoons extra-virgin olive oil
¼ cup finely chopped green onions

¼ cup dry white wine or fat-free low-sodium chicken broth
2 tablespoons lemon juice
2 tablespoons reduced-fat margarine
½ teaspoon salt
2 tablespoons chopped fresh parsley

NUTRIENTS PER SERVING:

¼ of total recipe
Calories: 210
Calories from fat: 39%
Protein: 19g
Total fat: 9g
Saturated fat: <1g
Cholesterol: 36mg
Carbohydrate: 10g
Dietary fiber: <1g
Sodium: 849mg
Dietary exchanges:
½ Starch, 3 Lean Meat

1. Combine flour, thyme, paprika, and red pepper in shallow dish; stir until well blended. Add scallops and toss until well coated. Shake off excess flour; set aside.

2. Heat oil in 12-inch nonstick skillet over medium high heat. Add scallops; cook 2 minutes. Turn scallops; cook 2 minutes or until opaque. Transfer scallops to serving platter; sprinkle with green onions.

3. Add wine and lemon juice to skillet. Bring to boil; boil 1 minute or until reduced slightly, scraping up browned bits from bottom and side. Remove from heat. Stir in margarine and salt until margarine is melted. Pour over scallops; sprinkle with parsley.

Makes 4 servings

SESAME SEEDS

These tiny seeds add a nutty, slightly sweet taste and delicate crunch to many dishes. Sesame seeds will boost the nutrient content, too.

BENEFITS:

Sesame seeds are low in calories but rich in beneficial minerals, including magnesium, calcium, and potassium, which help maintain healthy blood pressure. This is especially valuable to people with diabetes to help reduce their risks of heart disease and stroke. Among all nuts and seeds, sesame seeds have one of the largest amounts of cholesterol-lowering phytosterols, as well.

HOW TO SELECT AND STORE:

Sesame seeds come whole or hulled. Hulled seeds have had their outer shell removed and are usually white or light yellow. Unhulled, or whole, seeds retain their outer shell and can be brown, red, or black.

Sesame oil is available as plain or toasted and adds intense flavor to the foods it's cooked with. Store unhulled sesame seeds in an airtight container in a dry, cool, dark place. Hulled sesame seeds need to be stored in the refrigerator.

TIPS:

Sesame seeds are the main ingredient in tahini (sesame seed paste), which is a main component in hummus. You can add sesame seeds to homemade breads or muffins or sprinkle on steamed vegetables, stir-fries, or salads. Toasting sesame seeds intensifies their flavor. Try combining toasted sesame seeds with rice vinegar, tamari, and crushed garlic for a dressing for salads, vegetables, or noodles.

NUTRIENTS PER SERVING:

Sesame seeds, ½ ounce unhulled

Calories: 80
Protein: 2g
Total fat: 7g
Saturated fat: 1g
Cholesterol: 0mg
Carbohydrate: 4g
Dietary fiber: 2g
Sodium: 0mg
Potassium: 65mg
Calcium: 140mg
Iron: 2.1mg
Magnesium: 50mg
Copper: 0.4mg
Phosphorus: 90mg

SHRIMP

Although high in cholesterol, shrimp are naturally low in total fat and saturated fat, making them a good choice for anyone on a low-fat diet.

BENEFITS:

Shrimp are lean, high in protein, and rich in nutrients. They supply heart-healthy omega-3 fat, which is associated with a lower risk of heart disease, certain cancers, and eye diseases. Research also suggests omega-3s are important to cognitive function and may help lower elevated blood pressure. Although shrimp are rich in omega-3s, they are low in total fat compared to most complete protein sources. And they're very low in saturated fat. Shrimp also contain more heart-protective vitamin B_{12} and fewer calories, ounce for ounce, than other sources of animal protein.

HOW TO SELECT AND STORE:

Buy shrimp from a trusted source with a good reputation for having fresh seafood. Frozen shrimp keep for several weeks in the freezer. Fresh shrimp should be eaten within a day or two of purchase. Select fresh shrimp with firm bodies still attached to their shells and no black spots. Frozen shrimp should be tightly wrapped and stored in the freezer for up to one month.

TIPS:

Shrimp can be served as a main course or added to other dishes, such as soups, salads, stews, and stir-fries. Shrimp can be cooked with or without shells—follow recipe instructions. Frozen shrimp should be thawed in the refrigerator before cooking. To devein shrimp (optional), make a shallow cut along the rounded side and use the tip of a knife or your fingers to remove the black, string-like vein.

GRILLED TROPICAL SHRIMP

¼ cup barbecue sauce

2 tablespoons pineapple juice or orange juice

10 ounces medium shrimp in shells

2 medium firm nectarines

6 green onions, cut into 2-inch lengths, or yellow
  onion wedges

NUTRIENTS PER SERVING:

½ entire recipe
Calories: 232
Calories from fat: 7%
Protein: 25g
Total fat: 2g
Saturated fat: <1g
Cholesterol: 217mg
Carbohydrate: 30g
Dietary fiber: 3g
Sodium: 712mg
Dietary exchanges:
1½ Fruit, 2½ Lean Meat

1. Prepare grill for direct grilling. Stir together barbecue sauce and pineapple juice. Set aside.

2. Peel and devein shrimp. Cut each nectarine into 6 wedges. Thread shrimp, nectarines, and green onions onto 4 long metal skewers.

3. Spray grill grid with nonstick cooking spray. Grill skewers over medium coals 4 to 5 minutes or until shrimp are opaque, turning once and brushing frequently with barbecue sauce.

Makes 2 servings

SOY NUTS

Soy nuts are similar in texture and flavor to peanuts, but are much lower in fat and higher in protein. Soy nuts may taste sinful, but can be a guilt-free addition to a diabetes diet.

BENEFITS:

For people with diabetes, soy nuts are a great alternative to other nuts. Because soy nuts are generally lower in calories and fat, they're a better fit when you need to lose excess weight. And their larger protein and fiber loads make them easier on blood sugar. Plus, soy nuts have isoflavones, powerful phytonutrients that help fight heart disease, a common complication of diabetes. Soy nuts are also rich in potassium, which may help lower the elevated blood pressure that often accompanies diabetes.

HOW TO SELECT AND STORE:

Packaged soy nuts may be oil or dry roasted and salted or unsalted. Flavors may be added, such as barbeque or smoked flavorings. They also may be found covered in yogurt or chocolate. Store in a cool, dry place for up to six months. Once the package is opened, store in an airtight container.

NUTRIENTS PER SERVING:

Soy nuts, 1 ounce dry roasted without salt

Calories: 132
Protein: 10g
Total fat: 7g
Saturated fat: 1g
Cholesterol: 0mg
Carbohydrate: 9g
Dietary fiber: 5g
Sodium: 0mg
Potassium: 410mg
Calcium: 39mg
Iron: 1.1mg
Folate: 59mcg
Magnesium: 41mg
Vitamin E: <1mg

TIPS:

Soy nuts make a great snack alone or combined with fiber-packed cereals, dried fruit, and other nuts. They can be used as a crunchy topping for salads, too. To make soy nuts at home, soak dried soybeans in water for 6 to 8 hours, then drain and spread them in a single layer on an oiled baking sheet. Roast at 350°F for 30 to 50 minutes or until well browned, stirring often.

SPAGHETTI SQUASH

Diabetics can easily enjoy their favorite comfort food. Spaghetti squash is a great substitute for carbohydrate-rich pasta, as its flesh separates into spaghetti-like strands when cooked.

BENEFITS:

Although not as nutrient-rich as other winter squash, spaghetti squash has a place on a diabetic menu. It's a superb stand-in for regular pasta. It supplies far fewer calories, and it contains only about a third of the carbohydrates, so it has less effect on your blood sugar. Its fiber can keep you feeling full longer and works to lower blood cholesterol levels and even out blood sugar levels.

HOW TO SELECT AND STORE:

The peak season is from early fall through winter, though spaghetti squash are often available year-round. They are oblong and usually bright yellow in color. Choose squash that are hard and smooth with an even color. Avoid unripe greenish squash and those with bruises or signs of damage. Store uncut spaghetti squash at room temperature for several weeks.

NUTRIENTS PER SERVING:

Spaghetti squash, ½ cup cooked

Calories: 21
Protein: 1g
Total fat: 0g
Saturated fat: 0g
Cholesterol: 0mg
Carbohydrate: 5g
Dietary fiber: 1g
Sodium: 15mg
Potassium: 90mg
Calcium: 16mg
Iron: 0.3mg
Vitamin A: 85 IU
Vitamin C: 3mg
Folate: 6mcg

TIPS:

Cut the squash lengthwise and remove the seeds. Because it can be hard to cut a raw squash, you can briefly cook the whole squash in the microwave to help soften it. Cook until the flesh is tender and strands of squash are easily separated, 8 to 10 minutes in the microwave or 45 minutes to 1 hour in a 350°F oven. After cooking, remove and separate the spaghetti-like strands from the shell with a fork and serve with desired sauces and toppings.

SPINACH

Whether you eat it raw or cooked, spinach is a nutrition superstar that deserves a spot in a diabetic diet. However, cooked spinach is superior because it cooks down tremendously, making it an even more concentrated source of nutrients and fiber.

BENEFITS:

Spinach is reasonably high in fiber, offering twice as much as most other cooking or salad greens. Spinach fills you up and keeps you feeling full longer, a great advantage if you're pursuing weight loss. Spinach also contains the phytonutrient lipoic acid, which assists energy production and may help regulate blood sugar. Where spinach really shines is as a source of essential antioxidant vitamins A, C, and E and minerals manganese, selenium, and zinc.

HOW TO SELECT AND STORE:

Choose spinach with crisp, dark green leaves. Avoid limp or yellowing leaves. Refrigerate unwashed spinach in a loose plastic bag for three to four days. Prewashed bags of fresh spinach are readily available. Frozen or canned spinach is also a convenient option.

TIPS:

Raw spinach makes for a wonderful salad—either on its own or mixed with other leafy greens. Chopped raw spinach can be added to many different dishes to boost the nutrient contents, such as soups, sauces, casseroles, or chilis. To serve cooked spinach as a side, simmer the leaves in a small amount of water for about 5 minutes or until the leaves begin to wilt. Top with lemon juice, seasoned vinegar, sautéed garlic, or a dash of nutmeg.

STRAWBERRIES

Juicy strawberries make a great low-calorie, fiber-filled sweet that can stand in for high-calorie desserts and snacks.

BENEFITS:

Strawberries are rich in a variety of phytonutrients that protect the heart and assist in blood sugar control. Recent research found that the polyphenols in strawberries may have the ability to blunt a rise in blood sugar levels after consuming table sugar. Eating strawberries several times a week also appears to be associated with a lower risk of type 2 diabetes. Strawberries contain more vitamin C than oranges and grapefruit.

HOW TO SELECT AND STORE:

Look for plump strawberries that are ruby red, evenly colored, and have green, leafy tops. Avoid those that appear mushy or bruised. Bigger does not equal better. In fact, smaller strawberries tend to be the sweetest. Avoid strawberries in containers with juice stains or berries packed tightly with plastic wrap. Strawberries spoil quickly; it's best to serve them within a couple days of purchasing.

TIPS:

Though they are delicious on their own, strawberries can perk up several types of dishes. Add some sliced strawberries to your morning bowl of cereal or yogurt, to a spinach salad, or serve with pudding. You can add overripe strawberries to smoothies or fruit drinks or create a sauce for fruit salads or desserts. Add a splash of balsamic vinegar to bring out the sweet flavor of strawberries.

NUTRIENTS PER SERVING:

Strawberries, 1 cup halved raw

Calories: 49
Protein: 1g
Total fat: 0g
Saturated fat: 0g
Cholesterol: 0mg
Carbohydrate: 12g
Dietary fiber: 3g
Sodium: 0mg
Potassium: 235mg
Calcium: 24mg
Iron: 0.6mg
Vitamin A: 18 IU
Vitamin C: 89mg
Folate: 36mcg

CINNAMON TORTILLA WITH CREAM CHEESE & STRAWBERRIES

1 packet sugar substitute or equivalent
of 2 teaspoons sugar

⅛ teaspoon ground cinnamon

1 (6-inch) fat-free flour tortilla

Nonstick cooking spray

1 tablespoon reduced-fat soft cream cheese

⅓ cup fresh strawberry slices

1. Combine sugar substitute and cinnamon in cup; mix well. Heat large nonstick skillet over medium heat.

2. Lightly spray one side of tortilla with cooking spray; sprinkle with cinnamon mixture.

3. Place tortilla, cinnamon side down, in hot skillet. Cook 2 minutes or until lightly browned. Remove from skillet.

4. Spread uncooked side of tortilla with cream cheese; arrange strawberries down center of tortilla. Roll up tortilla and fold to serve.

Makes 1 serving

Tip: Use spreadable soft cream cheese for this recipe. Look for it in 8-ounce plastic containers in the dairy case.

NUTRIENTS PER SERVING:

Calories: 114
Calories from fat: 21%
Protein: 5g
Total fat: 3g
Saturated fat: 2g
Cholesterol: 8mg
Carbohydrate: 18g
Dietary fiber: 7g
Sodium: 256mg
Dietary exchanges:
½ Fruit, 1 Starch, ½ Fat

SUNFLOWER SEEDS

Sunflower seeds are a tasty gift from the beautiful sunflower. The kernels provide an array of protective nutrients.

BENEFITS:

Sunflower seeds are an excellent source of vitamin E, an essential vitamin that helps protect the heart and reduce the risk of diabetic complications. The phytosterols in sunflower seeds are natural cholesterol-lowering compounds and a good source of blood pressure-lowering magnesium, both of which are important for those with diabetes who also suffer from heart disease. Sunflower seeds contain mostly unsaturated fat, which can further lower cholesterol, especially when replacing saturated fat in other snacks.

HOW TO SELECT AND STORE:

Sunflower seeds are sold shelled or unshelled, salted or unsalted, and dry or oil roasted. For less fat and sodium, choose dry roasted, unsalted seeds. When buying unshelled seeds, look for firm, clean, unbroken shells. When purchasing shelled seeds, avoid those that appear yellowish. Sunflower seeds are prone to rancidity. They should be stored in an airtight container in the refrigerator or freezer.

NUTRIENTS PER SERVING:

Sunflower seeds (kernels), ½ ounce dry roasted without salt

Calories: 82
Protein: 3g
Total fat: 7g
Saturated fat: 0.5g
Cholesterol: 0mg
Carbohydrate: 3g
Dietary fiber: 1.5g
Sodium: 0mg
Potassium: 120mg
Calcium: 10mg
Iron: 0.5mg
Vitamin A: 1 IU
Vitamin E: 3.7mg
Folate: 34mcg

TIPS:

Sunflower seeds can lend crunch and flavor to green salads, tuna or chicken salad, stir-fries, or dips. Sprinkle them on hot and cold cereals or use them to make your own energy bars or trail mix. They also work well when baked in muffins, cookies, breads, or rolls.

SWEET POTATOES

This tiny tuber shouldn't only be eaten at Thanksgiving. Rich in flavor and nutrients, sweet potatoes have much to offer in a diabetic diet.

BENEFITS:

The carotenoids in sweet potatoes appear to help stabilize blood sugar levels due to their ability to lower insulin resistance by making cells more responsive to the hormone.

These effects not only aid in disease management, but also make it easier to drop the excess pounds. Sweet potatoes also offer fiber to keep you full for hours. The hefty nutrient profile can help protect your heart and the rest of your body from damage and complications related to diabetes. They supply infection-fighting vitamin C and blood pressure-lowering potassium.

NUTRIENTS PER SERVING:

Sweet potatoes, ½ cup baked
Calories: 90
Protein: 2g
Total fat: 0g
Saturated fat: 0g
Cholesterol: 0mg
Carbohydrate: 21g
Dietary fiber: 3.5g
Sodium: 35mg
Potassium: 475mg
Calcium: 38mg
Iron: 0.7mg
Vitamin A: 19,218 IU
Vitamin C: 20mg
Folate: 6mcg

HOW TO SELECT AND STORE:

Though often called a yam, a sweet potato is a different vegetable. Look for sweet potatoes that are small to medium in size with smooth, unbruised skin. Sweet potatoes are quite fragile and spoil easily. Any cut or bruise on the surface quickly spreads, ruining the whole potato. Store potatoes at room temperature.

TIPS:

To prepare sweet potatoes, boil unpeeled potatoes or bake or microwave them whole. Leaving the peel intact prevents excessive loss of precious nutrients and locks in its natural sweetness. Try sweet potatoes mashed, roasted, or in a soufflé. Use them to add moistness, flavor, and a boon of nutrients to quick breads or muffins.

SWISS CHARD

This leafy vegetable, with its crinkly green leaves and celery-like stalks, may offer unique benefits for blood sugar regulation.

BENEFITS:

An array of phytonutrients in Swiss chard may play a role in blocking the breakdown of carbohydrates into sugars, helping prevent blood sugar from spiking following meals. The fiber and protein in Swiss chard also help keep blood sugar more even by regulating the speed of digestion. And Swiss chard is loaded with antioxidant nutrients, including vitamins A and C, which help protect the body's cells from stress and inflammation.

HOW TO SELECT AND STORE:

Swiss chard is available year-round but is best in summer. The leaves may either be smooth or curly, while the stalks and veins range in color from red to yellow to creamy white. Look for leaves that are deep green without any browning or yellowing. Stalks should be crisp and without blemishes. Store in a sealed plastic bag in the refrigerator for up to five days. You can also blanch the leaves and then freeze them.

TIPS:

Wash Swiss chard under running water just before cooking. Stack the leaves and slice until you reach the stems. Only the white stems are tender enough to eat. Cut stems into half-inch slices, discarding the bottom. To bring out the sweetness, boil the leaves and stems and then use in almost any dish, including pasta, omelets, frittatas, and soups. Or simply enjoy it as a side dish, sautéed with olive oil, lemon juice, and garlic.

NUTRIENTS PER SERVING:

Swiss chard, ½ cup cooked
Calories: 18
Protein: 2g
Total fat: 0g
Saturated fat: 0g
Cholesterol: 0mg
Carbohydrate: 4g
Dietary fiber: 2g
Sodium: 155mg
Potassium: 480mg
Calcium: 51mg
Iron: 2.0mg
Vitamin A: 5,358 IU
Vitamin C: 16mg
Folate: 8mcg

TANGERINES

Tangerines are intensely sweet and juicy and pass easily as a dessert or treat, making them great for people with diabetes. Try the closely related clementine if you want to skip the seeds.

BENEFITS:

Tangerines are wonderfully sweet, yet supply only 47 calories and 12 grams of carbohydrate apiece, so they're a great substitute for typical treats, which are often loaded with calories, fats, and carbohydrates. Plus, tangerines are a decent source of soluble fiber to help stabilize blood sugar and lower blood cholesterol levels. And while tangerines contain a third as much vitamin C and folate as oranges, they provide three times the disease-fighting vitamin A.

HOW TO SELECT AND STORE:

This loose-skinned fruit is at its peak from November through June. Other varieties of mandarin oranges include the clementine, Satsuma orange, and honey tangerine. Most of the canned mandarin oranges are the Satsuma variety. Choose fresh tangerines that feel heavy for their size with smooth, unblemished skin. They should feel soft but not mushy. Store in the refrigerator for up to a week.

NUTRIENTS PER SERVING:

Tangerine, 1 medium raw
Calories: 47
Protein: 1g
Total fat: 0g
Saturated fat: 0g
Cholesterol: 0mg
Carbohydrate: 12g
Dietary fiber: 1.5g
Sodium: 0mg
Potassium: 145mg
Calcium: 33mg
Iron: 0.1mg
Vitamin A: 599 IU
Vitamin C: 24mg
Folate: 14mcg

TIPS:

Tangerines and other mandarins are great on their own or for other uses, like in salads. Just peel the fruit, separate the segments, and pull off the membrane from the segments, if desired. Be sure to remove the seeds. Try adding tangerine segments to coleslaw or tuna salad. Tangerine juice is a great in salad dressings and marinades.

TEA

Whether iced or hot, tea is the most popular beverage worldwide. Its popularity is partly due to the discovery of an array of potential health benefits. People with diabetes can indulge in this popular beverage without feeling guilty.

BENEFITS:

Drinking 2 to 3 cups of tea a day could offer several benefits to people with diabetes. Research shows that compounds in tea may improve the activity of insulin, potentially resulting in lower blood sugar. And antioxidants in tea may play a role in warding off diabetes complications, including cataracts and heart disease. Studies also suggest that tea may help suppress the growth of harmful bacteria that can cause infections, to which people with diabetes are more susceptible.

NUTRIENTS PER SERVING:

Tea (black), 1 cup brewed
Calories: 2
Protein: 0g
Total fat: 0g
Saturated fat: 0g
Cholesterol: 0mg
Carbohydrate: 1g
Dietary fiber: 0g
Sodium: 5mg
Potassium: 90mg
Iron: 0.1mg
Folate: 12mcg

HOW TO SELECT AND STORE:

All teas (except herbal) come from the leaves, stems, and buds of the Camellia Sinensis plant. The difference is in how they are processed. White tea is derived from the new leaves in early spring. Green tea is from leaves that are dried right after harvesting. Black and oolong teas are partially dried, crushed, and fermented to varying degrees. All types come either loose or in tea bags and should be stored in a cool, dark place. Be aware that instant, bottled, and herbal teas do not offer the same health benefits.

TIPS:

White and green teas should be brewed at a lower temperature (175°F) than oolong and black teas (195°F). For the best flavor and maximum nutritional benefits, steep tea for 3 to 5 minutes. Honey, sugar, lemon, or milk enhance flavor, but also add calories.

TEMPEH

Although tempeh may be bland in flavor, this versatile soybean by-product can aid in diabetes management.

BENEFITS:

Tempeh is a fermented soy food and an excellent substitute for higher-fat meats. It offers high quality protein but is lower in calories and saturated fat. Some research suggests soy products may help lower blood sugar levels. Additionally, soy products have been found to be easier on the vulnerable kidneys than animal protein. Soy protein also appears to help lower levels of damaging LDL cholesterol. And soy's isoflavones and other phytonutrients have been linked to a reduced risk of heart disease.

HOW TO SELECT AND STORE:

Tempeh is typically sold in natural food stores and in some supermarkets. Tempeh comes in many forms—precooked or uncooked, plain soy tempeh or soy-grain combinations, seasoned or unseasoned. Look for tempeh with a thin whitish bloom, with no pink, yellow, or blue coloration. Uncooked tempeh can keep in the refrigerator up to ten days or in the freezer for several months. Tempeh is usually purchased in a brick-like form and can be sliced similarly to tofu.

TIPS:

Tempeh's fairly bland taste allows it to absorb other flavors. Use crumbled tempeh if you want it as a background player and sliced if you want it as a featured ingredient. You can steam, bake, or broil tempeh. Try adding it to chili, pasta sauce, or grilled kebabs.

NUTRIENTS PER SERVING:

Tempeh, ½ cup cooked
Calories: 163
Protein: 15g
Total fat: 9g
Saturated fat: 3g
Monounsaturated fat: 3g
Cholesterol: 0mg
Carbohydrate: 8g
Dietary fiber: 4g
Sodium: 12mg
Calcium: 80mg
Potassium: 333mg
Magnesium: 64mg
Phosphorus: 210mg
Iron: 2mg
Zinc: 1mg
Vitamin B$_6$: 0.2mg
Vitamin B$_{12}$: 0.1mcg
Copper: 448mcg

TOMATOES

Tomatoes add color, flavor, and texture to every kind of dish. This sweet super food is easy for people with diabetes to enjoy every day.

BENEFITS:

Tomatoes are low in calories and fat free. The vitamin C in tomatoes is an antioxidant that supports healthy immune function. Their beta-carotene and other carotenoids are powerful weapons against heart disease, which is of particular importance to people with diabetes. And the antioxidant lycopene, which makes tomatoes red, may help reduce the risk of cardiovascular disease. Tomatoes also offer a good dose of potassium, which works to maintain healthy blood pressure.

HOW TO SELECT AND STORE:

Tomatoes come in a range of cheery colors—bright red, yellow, striped with yellow or green, even almost black. Real tomato taste comes only in season. Fortunately, canned tomatoes are ready to use any time and are nutritionally close to fresh. The best way to choose fresh tomatoes is by nose—if they have no aroma, they won't have any taste either. Don't store fresh tomatoes in the refrigerator as it ruins their taste and texture.

NUTRIENTS PER SERVING:

Tomato, 1 medium
Calories: 22
Protein: 1g
Total fat: 0g
Saturated fat: 0g
Cholesterol: 0mg
Carbohydrate: 5g
Dietary fiber: 1.5g
Sodium: 5mg
Potassium: 290mg
Calcium: 12mg
Iron: 0.3mg
Vitamin A: 1,025 IU
Vitamin C: 17mg
Folate: 18mcg

TIPS:

Try different colors and varieties of tomatoes for taste and eye appeal. Tomatoes are delicious raw on salads, on sandwiches, or on their own with a sprinkling of sea salt and herbs. They're also a great addition to many cooked dishes, such as stews, chilis, and pasta sauces. Roasting tomatoes concentrates their flavor.

TUNA

Canned tuna may be one of the most commonly consumed fish, but don't miss out on the wonderful flavor and meatlike texture of fresh tuna.

BENEFITS:

Tuna is a super source of protein, and a great way to get the omega-3 fats that experts recommend everyone get at least twice a week. Omega-3s can help fight the increased risk of cardiovascular disease that comes with diabetes. The omega-3 polyunsaturated fats in tuna help protect the heart by preventing erratic heart rhythms, making blood less likely to clot inside arteries, improving the ratio of "good" HDL cholesterol to "bad" LDL cholesterol, and promoting healthy blood pressure.

NUTRIENTS PER SERVING:

Tuna (canned in water), 3 ounces

Calories: 109
Protein: 20g
Total fat: 2.5g
Saturated fat: 0.5g
Cholesterol: 36mg
Carbohydrate: 0g
Dietary fiber: 0g
Sodium: 40mg
Potassium: 200mg
Calcium: 12mg
Iron: 0.8mg
Selenium: 56mcg
Phosphorus: 184mg
Vitamin B$_{12}$: 1mcg

HOW TO SELECT AND STORE:

Canned tuna may be packed in water, broth, or oil. Choose water-packed tuna. Fresh tuna is available as steaks, fillets, or pieces. Common varieties of tuna include yellowfin, which is deep red in color, and albacore, which is pale pink. Canned tunas usually indicate that it is either light tuna (usually yellowfin) or white tuna (albacore). Fresh tuna should be used within a day or two, or it can be kept frozen, tightly wrapped, for up to a month.

TIPS:

Lighten up tuna salad by using fresh lemon juice, olive oil, and a little mustard in place of mayonnaise. Consider nutrition-filled add-ins, such as leeks, fennel, peppers, carrots, fruit, and nuts. Fresh tuna steaks can be marinated and grilled or broiled for a tasty main dish or over a mixed green salad.

TURKEY BREAST

Lean and rich in protein, turkey breast no longer needs to be served just at Thanksgiving dinner or restricted from a diabetic's diet.

BENEFITS:

Skinless turkey breast is among the leanest of meats, giving people with diabetes a calorie-efficient way to get high quality protein with little saturated fat. Turkey breast is actually lower in fat than chicken. Turkey breast also contributes essential vitamins and minerals, including potassium for healthy blood pressure and zinc to promote wound healing and immune health.

HOW TO SELECT AND STORE:

Rather than buying a whole turkey, look for packages of breast meat. Feel free to prepare it with the skin on, which will lock in the juices and is also less expensive. Ground turkey breast is an option, but you'll want to read the label carefully as some ground turkey products also include dark meat, which will be higher in calories and fat. Turkey breast luncheon meat is lean and convenient. Store wrapped fresh turkey in the coldest section of your refrigerator and use within two to three days. Turkey breast can also be kept frozen.

NUTRIENTS PER SERVING:

Turkey breast, 3 ounces roasted skinless

Calories: 115
Protein: 26g
Total fat: 0.6g
Saturated fat: 0.2g
Cholesterol: 71mg
Carbohydrate: 0g
Dietary fiber: 0g
Sodium: 44mg
Potassium: 248mg
Zinc: 1.5mg
Iron: 1.3mg
Vitamin B$_{12}$: 0.3mcg
Vitamin B$_6$: 0.5mg
Selenium: 27mcg

TIPS:

To keep lean turkey breast moist, cook it with the skin and remove it before eating. Turkey breast can be grilled, roasted, or baked. It's done when the internal temperature reaches 160°F. Ground turkey breast is a great substitute for ground beef in burgers, chilis, meat loaves, tacos, and virtually any other recipe.

HERBED TURKEY BREAST WITH ORANGE SAUCE

1 large onion, chopped

3 cloves garlic, minced

1 teaspoon dried rosemary

½ teaspoon black pepper

1 boneless turkey breast (2 to 3 pounds)

1½ cups orange juice

Fresh rosemary sprigs (optional)

NUTRIENTS PER SERVING:

About 4 ounces turkey (cooked weight) with ⅓ cup sauce

Calories: 203
Protein: 36g
Total fat: 1g
Saturated fat: <1g
Cholesterol: 99mg
Carbohydrate: 10g
Fiber: 1g
Sodium: 70mg
Dietary exchanges:
½ Fruit, ½ Vegetable, 4 Lean Meat

1. Place onion in slow cooker. Combine garlic, rosemary, and pepper in small bowl; set aside.

2. Cut slices about three-fourths of the way through turkey at 2-inch intervals. Rub garlic mixture between slices.

3. Place turkey, cut side up, in slow cooker. Pour orange juice over turkey.

4. Cover; cook on low 7 to 8 hours. Serve turkey with sauce and fresh rosemary, if desired.

Makes 6 servings

WALNUTS

Compared to other nuts, walnuts provide the most omega-3 fats. Eating a handful of them daily is a delicious way to battle diabetes.

BENEFITS:

Eaten in moderation, walnuts are especially helpful for people with type 2 diabetes. They've been shown to reduce insulin resistance, excess body weight, and increased risk of heart disease. Walnuts provide a hefty amount of alpha-linolenic acid, the plant-based source of omega-3 fats that helps prevent blood clotting, reduce inflammation, and lower triglyceride levels in the blood. Walnuts also supply protein and soluble fiber, a combination of nutrients that helps to satisfy hunger, lower cholesterol, and smooth out blood sugar fluctuations.

HOW TO SELECT AND STORE:

Walnuts are available with or without the shell. Look for walnut shells without cracks or stains. Shelled walnuts are available whole, chopped, or ground and should be crisp rather than limp or rubbery. Check the freshness date before buying them. Store shelled walnuts in the refrigerator to prevent rancidity. In the shell, walnuts can be stored in a cool, dry place for up to a year.

NUTRIENTS PER SERVING:

Walnuts, 1 ounce dry roasted without salt
Calories: 185
Protein: 4g
Total fat: 18.5g
Saturated fat: 1.5g
Cholesterol: 0mg
Carbohydrate: 4g
Dietary fiber: 2g
Sodium: 0mg
Potassium: 125mg
Calcium: 28mg
Iron: 0.8mg
Folate: 28mcg
Magnesium: 45mg
Vitamin E: 0.2 mg

TIPS:

Walnuts can be enjoyed out of hand or added to many different foods. Roasting walnuts brings out the flavor. Add them to homemade granola or use them to top oatmeal, cereal, yogurt, and salads. Use them in muffins, pancakes, quick breads, and cookies.

WATER CHESTNUTS

With its skin on, the water chestnut looks like a regular chestnut that's fallen from a tree. But in actuality, the water chestnut is a crunchy, juicy tuberous vegetable that comes from a water plant.

BENEFITS:

This unassuming vegetable adds a hint of sweetness for very few calories to a variety of Asian-inspired dishes. The water chestnut's fiber and protein help counter the blood sugar-raising effects of its carbohydrates—an obvious plus for people with diabetes—and makes dishes that contain it more satisfying. Water chestnuts are also very low in sodium and a good source of potassium and magnesium, two minerals that help to regulate blood pressure.

HOW TO SELECT AND STORE:

Water chestnuts are available fresh in most Asian markets. Choose those that are firm with no signs of shriveling. They should be stored tightly wrapped in the refrigerator and used within one week. Peel off their brownish-black skin before using raw or cooked. Canned water chestnuts are readily available either sliced or whole. Be sure to rinse canned varieties before cooking to get rid of any excess sodium.

TIPS:

A staple in many Asian cuisines, water chestnuts are most often used in stir-fries; however, they have many other uses. Add them to salads for an extra crunch. Or chop them and add to tuna or chicken salads or veggie dips. Try them cooked with vegetables, such as asparagus or green beans. Wrap whole water chestnuts with turkey bacon.

NUTRIENTS PER SERVING:

Water chestnuts, ½ cup raw
Calories: 60
Protein: 1g
Total fat: 0g
Saturated fat: 0g
Cholesterol: 0mg
Carbohydrate: 15g
Dietary fiber: 2g
Sodium: 9mg
Potassium: 362mg
Calcium: 7mg
Phosphorus: 39mg
Magnesium: 14mg
Vitamin C: 3mg
Folate: 10mcg

WHEAT BRAN

Literally bursting with fiber, wheat bran—the hard outer shell of the wheat kernel—offers an easy way to boost the fiber in almost anything you eat.

BENEFITS:

Wheat bran is a great tool for increasing fiber intake as it can easily be incorporated into several foods. And for people with diabetes, eating a fiber-rich diet, filled with whole grains, fruits, and vegetables, is essential in keeping blood sugar in a healthier range. Fiber-rich foods play an important role in weight loss, too, which is important for those with diabetes who need to lose weight to improve their condition. Wheat bran also contributes heart-protective nutrients, such as niacin, which boosts HDL ("good") cholesterol levels, and potassium and magnesium, which help lower blood pressure.

HOW TO SELECT AND STORE:

Wheat bran is usually available in bulk bins in the natural foods section of the supermarket, or it may be found with grains or cereals. Wheat bran is best stored in airtight containers in the refrigerator for prolonged shelf life.

NUTRIENTS PER SERVING:

Wheat bran, ½ cup
Calories: 63
Protein: 5g
Total fat: 1g
Saturated fat: 0g
Cholesterol: 0mg
Carbohydrate: 19g
Dietary fiber: 12g
Sodium: 0mg
Potassium: 345mg
Magnesium: 177mg
Iron: 3.1mg
Zinc: 2.1mg
Niacin: 3.9mg
Vitamin B$_6$: 0.4mg

TIPS:

Wheat bran can be added to many foods to boost fiber content. Sprinkle it over hot or cold cereals or on yogurt or applesauce. Add wheat bran to recipes for breads, cookies, muffins, and pancakes. It can easily be added to ground meat dishes, such as meat loaves, burgers, or casseroles. Toasting wheat bran gives it an especially nutty flavor and crunchy texture.

YELLOW SQUASH

A type of summer squash, yellow squash is also known as crookneck squash because of its swan-like neck.

BENEFITS:

Yellow squash's thin edible skin, tender seeds, small stock of carbohydrates, and high water content together aid in diabetes control, helping to keep post-meal blood sugar levels from spiking, and providing a fullness that can make it easier to skip seconds. Yellow squash also contains vitamin C and beta-carotene, antioxidants that may play a role in fighting heart disease. It is also rich in folate, which appears to lower the level of homocysteine, a substance that can damage blood vessels. The vitamin C can fight inflammation.

HOW TO SELECT AND STORE:

Yellow squash is at its peak during summer months but is available year-round. It should feel heavy for its size and have shiny, unblemished skin. Look for summer squash that is small to average in size. Larger yellow squash may have harder skin and tend to have larger seeds and stringy flesh. It is very perishable and should be stored unwashed in a plastic bag in the refrigerator for up to five days.

TIPS:

Wash yellow squash under cool running water and then cut off both ends. It can be sliced into rounds and enjoyed raw with a dip or sliced or grated into thin strips and added to a fresh salad. Sauté yellow squash with onions, sweet bell peppers, eggplant, and tomatoes, to make the delicious side dish ratatouille.

NUTRIENTS PER SERVING:

Yellow squash, ½ cup cooked
Calories: 21
Protein: 1g
Total fat: 0g
Saturated fat: 0g
Cholesterol: 0mg
Carbohydrate: 3g
Dietary fiber: 1g
Sodium: 0mg
Potassium: 160mg
Calcium: 20mg
Iron: 0.3mg
Vitamin A: 1,005 IU
Vitamin C: 10mg
Folate: 21mcg

YOGURT

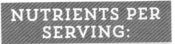

Yogurt has a hefty nutrient profile and can be enjoyed in several ways, making it an ally in diabetes management.

Yogurt, 1 cup plain low-fat
Calories: 154
Protein: 13g
Total fat: 4g
Saturated fat: 2.5g
Cholesterol: 15mg
Carbohydrate: 17g
Dietary fiber: 0g
Sodium: 170mg
Potassium: 575mg
Calcium: 448mg
Iron: 0.2mg
Vitamin A: 125 IU
Vitamin C: 2mg
Folate: 27mcg

BENEFITS:

Yogurt is great for people with diabetes. It's a nutrient-rich substitute for higher-calorie sugary desserts and provides satisfying protein to help battle hunger and even out blood sugar. The protein content in yogurt allows it to be used easily in meals as a substitute for high-fat meats. And the live active bacteria cultures found in most yogurt help with digestive health by suppressing the growth of harmful bacteria in the intestinal tract. These beneficial bacteria promote immune health, too. Stronger immune function may help counter the increased vulnerability to infections that comes with diabetes.

HOW TO SELECT AND STORE:

To keep fat and calories low, look for low-fat or nonfat yogurt. The addition of fruit or sweeteners adds calories, so look for plain varieties and add your own flavorings. Some yogurt products are sweetened with noncaloric sweeteners. Yogurt will keep for up to ten days past the "sell by" date.

TIPS:

Yogurt makes a great portable meal or snack on its own, but it has several other great uses. Yogurt makes a wonderful base for smoothies when blended with fresh fruit and juice. Or top your morning bowl of cereal with yogurt instead of milk. Yogurt works as a great substitute in recipes that call for high-fat ingredients like cream or sour cream. And yogurt is especially well suited as a base for dips and salad dressings.

ZUCCHINI

Often mistaken for a cucumber, zucchini, a type of summer squash, has a high water content that makes it one of the lowest-calorie vegetables you'll find.

BENEFITS:

With so little carbohydrate to spark a jump in blood sugar levels, zucchini gets an invitation to join its cousin, the yellow squash, as welcome regulars in a diabetic diet. Zucchini provides folate, an essential B vitamin, and generous doses of vitamins A and C, all of which can help protect the heart and blood vessels from cell damage that may lead to cardiovascular disease, a common diabetes complication. And zucchini's fiber can play a role in lowering elevated blood cholesterol levels, while its potassium can help maintain a steady heartbeat and keep blood pressure in check.

NUTRIENTS PER SERVING:

Zucchini, ½ cup cooked
Calories: 14
Protein: 1g
Total fat: 0g
Saturated fat: 0g
Cholesterol: 0mg
Carbohydrate: 2g
Dietary fiber: 1g
Sodium: 0mg
Potassium: 240mg
Calcium: 16mg
Iron: 0.3mg
Vitamin A: 1,005 IU
Vitamin C: 12mg
Folate: 25mcg

HOW TO SELECT AND STORE:

Zucchini is available year-round in most supermarkets. Look for smaller squash, about six to nine inches long, for the best flavor. The skin should be deep green or yellow, and it should be firm and unblemished. Zucchini should be stored in the refrigerator and used within a few days.

TIPS:

The mild flavor of zucchini complements other ingredients in a variety of dishes. It is especially delicious sautéed with tomatoes and onions. Zucchini makes a tasty and nutritious addition to vegetable lasagna, marinara sauce, or stir-fries. The perfect way to use a larger zucchini is to grate it and bake it into low-fat cakes or quick breads—adding nutrition and moistness without any detectable flavor.

GLOSSARY

AMINO ACIDS: the building blocks of protein. Twenty amino acids are necessary to help the body grow, repair itself, and fight disease. Nine of these are considered essential because they must come from food you eat, while the body can produce the others.

ANTHOCYANINS: a type of flavonoid responsible for the red and blue pigments found in certain fruits and vegetables. Anthocyanins can help prevent the growth of cancer, lower LDL "bad" cholesterol, and prevent clots from forming.

ANTIOXIDANTS: certain vitamins, minerals, and enzymes that help protect cells from damage caused by oxidation, which can result from exposure to tobacco smoke, sunlight, radiation, and pollution, as well as aging and illness. Antioxidants offer protection against heart disease, cancer, diabetes, eye disease, and numerous other health problems.

BETA-CAROTENE: a potent antioxidant found in red, orange, and yellow plant foods and in some dark green vegetables. It is converted to vitamin A in the body.

CARBOHYDRATE: one of the three main nutrients in food, providing 4 calories per gram. Complex carbohydrates are the primary supplier of energy in the diet and can be found mainly in breads, cereals, pasta, potatoes, squash, beans, and peas. Sugars are also known as simple carbohydrates and provide calories (and energy) with few nutrients.

CAROTENOIDS: pigments that give produce their red, orange, and yellow colors. Over 600 different carotenoids have been identified, some of which are powerful antioxidants, including beta-carotene, lutein, and lycopene.

CHOLESTEROL: a waxy substance produced by the liver that is part of every cell in the body. The body uses it to manufacture hormones, bile acid, and other essential substances. It is also supplied by the diet when you eat foods from animal sources. Some cholesterol is essential for life, but it can be dangerous as it builds up on artery walls, narrowing blood vessels. LDL (low density lipoprotein), or "bad," cholesterol deposits cholesterol in blood vessels, where it forms plaque that can lead to heart disease. HDL (high density lipoprotein), or "good," cholesterol helps remove cholesterol from the blood and delivers it to the liver, where it can be eliminated.

CRUCIFEROUS VEGETA-BLES: a family of vegetables, which includes bok choy, broccoli, brussels sprouts, cabbage, cauliflower, kale, mustard greens, and turnips, that has cancer-fighting properties. The family is named for its cross-shaped flowers.

DIABETIC RETINOPATHY: damage to the retina of the eye that results from poorly controlled blood sugar levels. It can lead to severe vision loss or even blindness.

EXCHANGE LISTS: lists of foods grouped into categories, such as starches, vegetables, fruits, meats, and so on, with predetermined portion sizes. All food exchanges within a category have roughly equivalent nutritional value and impact on blood sugar levels.

FAT: one of the three major nutrients in food, providing 9 calories per gram. Saturated fats, found in butter, stick margarine, fats in meat, poultry skin, and whole-fat dairy foods, are solid at room temperature and can raise blood cholesterol levels. Unsaturated fats, found in vegetable oils, nuts, olives, and avocados, are liquid at room temperature and help lower blood cholesterol levels.

FIBER: the parts of plants that cannot be digested. Insoluble fiber absorbs water and adds bulk to stools, easing elimination, promoting digestive regularity, and providing a feeling of fullness after eating. Soluble fiber forms a gel in the digestive tract and slows the rate of digestion, which helps regulate blood sugar levels and prevent the absorption of cholesterol.

FLAVONOIDS: health-protective substances are found in the colorful skins of vegetables, fruits, and berries, as well as in beverages such as tea, red wine, and fruit juices. Their health benefits are similar to those of antioxidants.

"FREE FOOD": any food or drink that contains less than 20 calories or 5 grams or less of carbohydrates per serving. For people with diabetes, small amounts of these foods can be enjoyed with little or no effect on blood sugar levels.

GLUCOSE: the basic form of sugars and carbohydrates found in food. It is transported in the blood and used as the primary source of energy. Glucose in the blood is referred to as blood sugar.

GLYCEMIC INDEX (GI): a scale that ranks foods from 0 to 100 based on the rate at which different carbs are converted into blood glucose. Foods with a high GI score tend to be digested and converted into glucose the fastest.

IMMUNE FUNCTION: the body's ability to defend itself against disease and illness.

INSULIN: a hormone made by the body that helps transfer glucose from the blood into cells, where it can be used to fuel body functions.

INSULIN RESISTANCE: the diminished ability of cells to respond to insulin, which causes an increase in blood glucose levels. Insulin resistance forces the body to make more insulin in an attempt to transfer the excess glucose in the blood into the cells.

LEGUMES: edible seeds that grow in pods; includes beans, peas, lentils, and peanuts.

LUTEIN: a pigment found in foods that are bright yellow, orange, and green. Along with zeaxanthin, this carotenoid pigment is linked to a reduced risk of macular degeneration and cataracts.

LYCOPENE: a powerful antioxidant that lends red color to numerous foods and is especially abundant in tomatoes. It helps protect against prostate cancer, lung cancer, and heart disease.

MACULAR DEGENERATION: the deterioration of the central portion of the retina that causes severe vision loss and even blindness, most often in people over 60. Certain nutrients, including vitamins C, E, beta-carotene, zinc, and copper, can decrease the risk of vision loss.

METABOLIC SYNDROME: a combination of conditions, including high blood pressure, high blood sugar, too much fat around the waist, low HDL cholesterol, and high triglycerides, that tend to occur together and, when they do, increase the risk of type 2 diabetes, heart disease, and stroke.

OMEGA-3 FATS: a type of unsaturated fat essential for human health that is found in fish, including salmon, tuna, and halibut. They are also found other seafood, including algae and krill as well as in some plants and nut oils. These healthy fats play a critical role in brain function, as well as normal growth and development and they help to reduce inflammation that can lead to heart disease, cancer, and arthritis.

PECTIN: a soluble fiber that helps to lower artery-damaging LDL cholesterol. Pectin is found in most plants but is most abundant in apples, cranberries, plums, grapefruits, lemons, and oranges.

PLAQUE: the fatty substance that builds up in blood vessels. It can constrict blood flow and lead to heart attack and stroke.

PROTEIN: one of the three major nutrients found in food, providing 4 calories per gram. It helps with cell growth and repair as well as with fighting disease. Vegetable sources of protein include beans, nuts, and whole grains. Animal sources include fish, poultry, and meat.

PHYTOCHEMICALS: another name for phytonutrients.

PHYTONUTRIENTS: natural substances found in plants that help protect the plant from disease. In humans, phytonutrients have numerous health-promoting properties; they function as antioxidants to help rid the body of toxins and prevent inflammation.

POLYPHENOLS: natural chemicals in plants, including in fruits, vegetables, seeds, legumes, and grains, that are responsible for much of their color, flavor, and scent. They act as antioxidants and block enzymes that can promote cancer growth.

TRIGLYCERIDES: the name for fat that travels in your blood, where it is transported to cells and used for energy. High levels of triglycerides can raise your risk of heart disease and may be a sign of metabolic syndrome.

U.S. DIETARY GUIDELINES: official food and nutrition advice for Americans ages 2 and older, jointly published by the U.S. Department of Health and Human Services and the Food and Drug Administration. The guidelines are revised every 5 years, based on the latest scientific research on the effect of food and nutrients on health.

ZEAXANTHIN: a pigment found in foods that are bright yellow, orange, and green. Along with lutein, this pigment in the carotenoid family is linked to a reduced risk of macular degeneration and cataracts.